The Rise of Acid Reflux in Asia

Prateek Sharma · Shobna Bhatia
Khean Lee Goh
Editors

The Rise of Acid Reflux in Asia

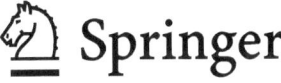

Editors
Prateek Sharma
University of Kansas School of
  Medicine, VA Medical Center
Kansas City, MO, USA

Shobna Bhatia
Gastroenterology
KEM Hospital
Mumbai, Maharashtra, India

Khean Lee Goh
University of Malaya
Kuala Lumpur, Malaysia

ISBN 978-81-322-0845-7   ISBN 978-81-322-0846-4   (eBook)
DOI 10.1007/978-81-322-0846-4

Library of Congress Control Number: 2017954939

Printed on acid-free paper

This Springer imprint is published by Springer Nature
The registered company is Springer (India) Pvt. Ltd.
The registered company address is: 7th Floor, Vijaya Building, 17 Barakhamba Road, New Delhi 110 001, India

Preface

Symptoms of gastroesophageal reflux disease (GERD), a very common occurrence in the adult Western population, were once considered uncommon in the Asian continent. However, with the "Westernization" of society in the east, GERD is now a common disorder in Asia and accounts for a large proportion of visits to the general practitioner and gastroenterologist.

How do we define GERD in Asia? How common is it? Why is GERD rising in Asia? What are the complications of GERD? And finally, how do we manage GERD in the Asian population? These are all questions that are becoming increasingly important given the changing epidemiology of GERD in this part of the globe. To answer some of these questions, we, the editors, have been fortunate to assemble the leading expert gastroenterologists from Asia to review the latest literature and provide their expertise on the approach to GERD in Asia.

We would like to thank the experts for uniformly providing succinct and state-of-the-art chapters, the publishers for believing in us regarding the importance of this topic, and our local institution research teams for their efforts.

Kansas City, MO, USA   Prateek Sharma
Mumbai, Maharashtra, India   Shobna Bhatia
Kuala Lumpur, Malaysia   Khean Lee Goh

Contents

Contributors

Philip Abraham Division of Gastroenterology, P.D. Hinduja Hospital, Mumbai, India

Rupa Banerjee Asian Institute of Gastroenterology, Hyderabad, India

Shobna Bhatia Gastroenterology, KEM Hospital, Mumbai, Maharashtra, India

Philip W.Y. Chiu Division of Upper GI and Metabolic Surgery, Department of Surgery, Institute of Digestive Disease, The Chinese University of Hong Kong, Hong Kong, SAR, China

Kwong Ming Fock Changi Hospital, National University of Singapore, Singapore, Singapore

Srinivas Gaddam Department of Gastroenterology and Hepatology, Veterans Affairs Medical Center, Kansas City, MO, USA

Khean Lee Goh University of Malaya, Kuala Lumpur, Malaysia

Deepak Kumar Gupta Department of Gastroenterology, Seth GS Medical College and KEM Hospital, Mumbai, India

Ken Haruma Department of General Internal Medicine 2, Kawasaki Medical School General Medical Center, Okayama, Japan

Khek Yu Ho National University of Singapore/National University Hospital, Singapore, Singapore

Michio Hongo Kurokawa General Hospital, Tohoku University, Kurokawa, Miyagi, Japan

Takashi Kondo Division of Gastroenterology, Department of Internal Medicine, Hyogo College of Medicine, Hyogo, Japan

Somchai Leelakusolvong Gastrointestinal Division, Department of Medicine, Siriraj Hospital, Bangkok, Thailand

Sally Wai Yin Luk Division of Upper GI and Metabolic Surgery, Department of Surgery, Institute of Digestive Disease, The Chinese University of Hong Kong, Hong Kong SAR, China

Varocha Mahachai Department of Gastroenterology, Chulalongkorn University, Bangkok, Thailand

Noriaki Manabe Division of Endoscopy and Ultrasonography, Department of Clinical Pathology and Laboratory Medicine, Kawasaki Medical School, Kurashiki, Japan

Hiroto Miwa Division of Gastroenterology, Department of Internal Medicine, Hyogo College of Medicine, Hyogo, Japan

Hardik Parikh Department of Gastroenterology, KEM Hospital and Seth GS Medical College, Mumbai, India

Duvvur Nageshwar Reddy Asian Institute of Gastroenterology, Hyderabad, India

Julius Carlo R. Rustia Gastroenterologist and Specialized Advanced Therapeutic Endoscopist, Aquinas University Hospital Foundation Inc, LegazpiCity, Albay, Philippines

Prateek Sharma University of Kansas School of Medicine, VA Medical Center, Kansas City, MO, USA

Prashanth Vennalaganti Department of Gastroenterology and Hepatology, University of Kansas School of Medicine, Kansas City, KS, USA

Ratha-korn Vilaichone Gastrointestinal Unit, Department of Medicine, Thammasat University Hospital, Pathumthani, Thailand

Justin Che-yeun Wu Department of Medicine & Therapeutics, S.H. Ho Centre for Digestive Health, Institute of Digestive Disease, Prince of Wales Hospital, Hong Kong, SAR, China

Takahisa Yamasaki Division of Gastroenterology, Department of Internal Medicine, Hyogo College of Medicine, Hyogo, Japan

Abbreviations

ACEI	Angiotensin converting enzyme inhibitor
ACG	American College of Gastroenterology
ACP	American College of Physicians
AFI	Autofluorescence imaging
ARS	Anti-reflux surgery
BE	Barrett's esophagus
cagA	Cytotoxin-associated gene A
CLE	Columnar-lined esophagus
CLE	Confocal endomicroscopy
DIS	Dilated intercellular spaces
EAC	Esophageal adenocarcinoma
EE	Erosive esophagitis
EGD	Esophagogastroduodenoscopy
ENT	Ear, nose, and throat
ERD	Erosive reflux disease
ESEM	Endoscopically suspected esophageal metaplasia
EST	Electrical stimulation therapy
ETMI	Endoscopic trimodal imaging
FEST	Far East Study
FSSG	Frequency scale for the symptoms of GERD
GER	Gastroesophageal reflux
GERD	Gastroesophageal reflux disease
GERQ	Gastroesophageal reflux questionnaire
GI	Gastrointestinal
GIS	Gastroesophageal reflux disease impact scale
GSRS	Gastrointestinal symptom rating scale
HGIN	High-grade intraepithelial neoplasia
H. pylori	*Helicobacter pylori*
HRME	High-resolution magnification endoscopy
HRQOL	Health-related quality of life
$H_2RA(s)$	Histamine$_2$ receptor antagonist(s)
IHC	Immunohistochemistry
IPCL	Intrapapillary capillary loop
LES	Lower esophageal sphincter

LIFS	Light-induced fluorescence spectroscopy
LPR	Laryngopharyngeal reflux
LSM	Lifestyle modification
MAO	Maximal acid output
MII	Multichannel intraluminal impedance
MNBI	Mean nocturnal baseline impedance
NAB	Nocturnal acid breakthrough
NAR	Non-acid reflux
NBI	Narrow-band imaging
NCCP	Non-cardiac chest pain
NERD	Non-erosive reflux disease
NHWS	National Health and Wellness Survey
NPV	Negative predictive value
OGJ	Esophagogastric junction
PEF	Peak expiratory flow
PNDS	Postnasal drip syndrome
PPI(s)	Proton pump inhibitor(s)
PPV	Positive predictive value
PSPW	Post-reflux swallow-induced peristaltic wave
QOL	Quality of life
QUEST	Questionnaire for diagnosis of reflux disease
RDQ	Reflux disease questionnaire
RF	Radio frequency
RFS	Reflux finding score
RSI	Reflux symptom index
SAP	Symptom-association probability
S-BEST	Sendai Barrett's Esophagus Study
SI	Symptom index
SSI	Symptom sensitivity index
SSRIs	Selective serotonin reuptake inhibitors
TCA	Tricyclic antidepressants
tLESR(s)	Transient lower esophageal sphincter relaxation(s)
WLE	White light endoscopy

Defining GERD in Asia: Different from the West?

Justin Che-yeun Wu

Abstract
The definition of GERD (gastroesophageal reflux disease) needs a combined approach that includes symptomatology, endoscopy, and reflux investigations. The Montreal classification has proposed an extensive coverage of various entities of GERD, which include esophageal and extraesophageal syndromes. The American College of Gastroenterology guidelines emphasize the role of endoscopy and reflux investigations to define GERD.

A global standardized definition of GERD is needed to evaluate better the epidemiological trends and facilitate conduction of clinical trials in the Asian population. However, defining GERD in Asia remains a challenge because of the vast multiethnic and multicultural nature, relatively low prevalence of GERD, and preponderance of *Helicobacter pylori*-related diseases in Asia. Typical reflux symptoms such as heartburn are poorly interpreted by Asian patients. Pretest probability of diagnostic tests for GERD is generally lower in Asia because of the low prevalence of GERD in particular extraesophageal syndromes. Because of the significant overlap of GERD and *H. pylori*-related diseases, diagnostic tests for *H. pylori* or prompt endoscopy prior to PPI test help avoid the misdiagnosis of peptic ulcer disease as GERD. Despite the objective nature of evaluation of reflux and its association with symptoms, reflux investigations are not readily accessible in Asia. Validation studies are needed to evaluate the role of reflux investigations for defining GERD in Asia.

Keywords
Asia • Definition • Gastroesophageal reflux disease • GERD • *Helicobacter pylori* • EndoscopyPPI

J.C.-y. Wu (✉)
Department of Medicine & Therapeutics, S.H. Ho Centre for Digestive Health, Institute of Digestive Disease, Prince of Wales Hospital, Hong Kong, SAR, China
e-mail: justinwu@cuhk.edu.hk

© Springer India 2018
P. Sharma et al. (eds.), *The Rise of Acid Reflux in Asia*,
DOI 10.1007/978-81-322-0846-4_1

1

Introduction

Gastroesophageal reflux disease (GERD) is a chronic relapsing acid-peptic disorder that is caused by the reflux of gastric content. It is a disease entity characterized by diverse spectrum of clinical presentations ranging from mild symptom to life-threatening complications. "Physiological" acid reflux occurs in normal people, and it is typically short-lived and asymptomatic. The diagnosis of GERD is applied only when there are symptoms, disturbance to normal life, or tissue damage related to reflux. Unfortunately, there is no single reliable "gold standard" diagnostic investigation for GERD since none has both good sensitivity and specificity. As a result, the definition of GERD is subject to variability in perception and interpretation of symptoms and investigations, evolving new concepts in pathophysiology and technology advances [1].

Defining GERD in Asia remains a challenging task. There is marked heterogeneity in definition due to the vast multiethnic and multicultural population in Asia. There may also be dynamism in risk factors and pathophysiologic mechanisms that contribute to the changing epidemiology of GERD in Asia [2–9]. Yet it is important to establish a universal definition of GERD that can be applied in Asia. First, it enables international epidemiological studies that help identify the specific risk factors and monitor the secular trend in Asian population. This will help develop strategies of disease prevention. Second, a universal definition of GERD facilitates the conduction of clinical trials for the development of GERD treatment in Asian patients [10–13] (Table 1.1).

Montreal Classification

The Montreal classification is the most widely used classification system for GERD. It consists of consensus statements on definition and classification of GERD based on systematic reviews of the literature and a modified Delphi approach [14]. The classification incorporates a pathophysiologic process and a symptom-based definition, which is defined as a condition that develops when the reflux of stomach contents causes troublesome symptoms and/or complications. The term

Table 1.1 Special features of definition of GERD in Asia

1.	Significant overlap of symptoms of GERD and *Helicobacter pylori*-related diseases
2.	Poor interpretation of heartburn as marker of GERD
3.	Discrepancy between definitions based on symptom frequency and quality of life impairment
4.	Undefined significance of extraesophageal syndromes
5.	Lower pretest probability of diagnostic tests because of low prevalence
6.	Endoscopy is important for exclusion of peptic ulcer and gastric cancer
7.	Concepts of "minimal change" esophagitis and peculiar definition of gastroesophageal junction which leads to different definition of Barrett's esophagus
8.	Limited access of reflux investigations such as pH and impedance monitoring

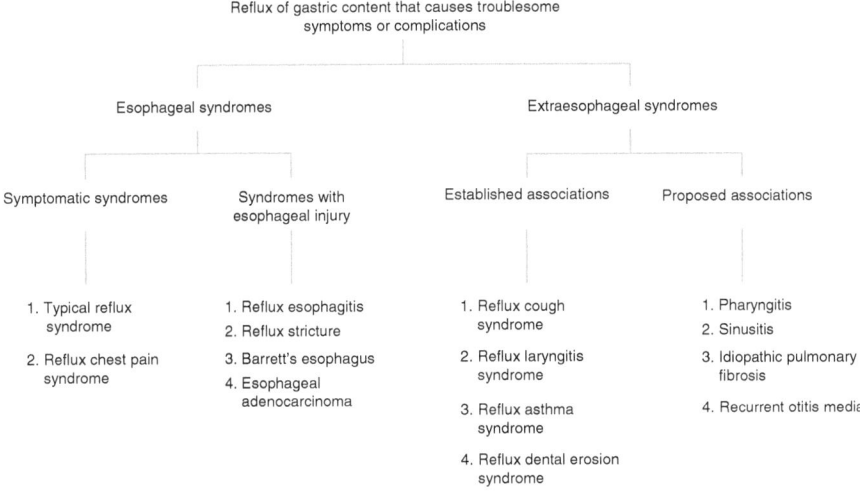

Fig. 1.1 Montreal classification of GERD

"troublesome" has been underscored in the definition because of its implication on the negative impact on the quality of life and morbid nature of the condition from a patient's perspective.

Compared to the other definitions, the Montreal classification is the preferred system because it adopts a more comprehensive and broader approach of defining GERD. Under this classification scheme, entities of atypical symptoms, asymptomatic esophagitis, and extraesophageal manifestations of GERD have been included. And it is broadly categorized into esophageal and extraesophageal syndromes (Fig. 1.1).

Esophageal Syndromes

The esophageal syndromes are further subclassified into symptomatic syndromes and syndromes with esophageal injury.

Symptomatic Reflux Syndromes

There are two symptomatic syndromes. The *typical reflux syndrome* is defined by the presence of troublesome heartburn and/or regurgitation. Heartburn is defined as a burning sensation in the retrosternal area (behind the breastbone), whereas regurgitation is defined as the feeling of upward flow of gastric refluxate into the mouth or hypopharynx. Typical reflux syndrome is a clinical diagnosis based on characteristic symptomatology rather than diagnostic tests. The Montreal classification proposes a symptom-frequency-based definition of GERD, which is defined as mild heartburn and/or regurgitation of at least 2 days per week or moderate/severe heartburn and/or regurgitation at least 1 day a week.

The *reflux chest pain syndrome* refers to the episodes of troublesome chest pain that is caused by gastroesophageal reflux. The chest pain mimics angina, which is not readily distinguishable from ischemic heart disease. The chest pain may or may not be accompanied with heartburn or regurgitation.

Syndromes with Esophageal Injury

The syndromes with esophageal injury refer to various entities of reflux-related tissue damage that can be detected endoscopically. *Reflux esophagitis* is the commonest syndrome with esophageal injury. It is defined by the presence of mucosal breaks at the distal esophagus adjacent to the gastroesophageal junction. Among the various endoscopic classification systems of reflux esophagitis, Los Angeles classification is by far the best validated system with good reproducibility and interobserver variation [15]. New image-enhancing endoscopic modalities, such as narrowband imaging, have been proposed for better definition of esophageal injury related to GERD [16–18]. However, these have not been included as routine measures for defining GERD, and their role is not clearly defined [19, 20].

The other entities of syndromes with esophageal injury in the Montreal classification include peptic stricture, Barrett's esophagus, and esophageal adenocarcinoma. Classically, Barrett's esophagus is defined as the presence of intestinal metaplasia in the biopsies of a segment of columnar-lined esophagus. In the Montreal classification, an intermediate term known as "endoscopically suspected esophageal metaplasia" (ESEM) has been suggested for endoscopic findings of columnar-lined esophagus that awaits confirmation by histologic examination. It is not uncommon that intestinal metaplasia may not be identified in the histologic examination despite the endoscopic finding that is compatible with Barrett's esophagus. The Montreal classification has therefore adopted a simplified definition of Barrett's esophagus primarily based on the presence of columnar epithelium in the esophagus with the presence or absence of intestinal metaplasia specified. Esophageal adenocarcinoma is the most severe form of reflux syndrome with esophageal injury. It is strongly associated with chronic reflux symptoms, male gender, and obesity in the Western population. It is generally believed that esophageal adenocarcinoma is the result of progression from Barrett's esophagus with dysplasia.

Extraesophageal Syndromes

The Montreal classification has also included a number of extraesophageal syndromes in the definition of GERD based on the epidemiological associations or biologically plausible mechanisms. The association between GERD and conditions such as chronic cough, chronic laryngitis, asthma, and dental erosions is supported largely by cross-sectional observational studies. However, the results on the efficacy of acid-suppressive therapy in the treatment of these diseases have been conflicting. These observations suggest that GERD may only be one of the risk factors that contribute to the occurrence of these disease entities. Other extraesophageal syndromes, which include pharyngitis, sinusitis, idiopathic pulmonary fibrosis, and recurrent otitis media, have been proposed. However, the strength of evidence that supports the association between these conditions and GERD is weak.

There are several highlights of Montreal classification that justify its position as the preferred definition of GERD. First, the classification focuses on well-documented pathophysiologic process and symptoms reported by patients for the definition. Despite the major advances in esophageal pH and impedance testing, as well as improved sensitivity of endoscopic detection of reflux-related mucosal damage, there is still a lack of gold standard diagnostic investigations of GERD. The Montreal classification is relatively independent of these technological advances so as to obviate the need of frequent revision in the definition. Second, the classification has an extensive coverage of all possible syndromes that are related to GERD. These syndromes include a considerable subgroup of GERD patients who are asymptomatic, yet they have complications such as severe erosive esophagitis or Barrett's esophagus [21]. It also highlights the importance of extraesophageal or atypical presentation of GERD.

ACG Guidelines

The guidelines published by the American College of Gastroenterology (ACG) addressed the limited accuracy of symptom-based diagnosis and empiric PPI (proton pump inhibitor) therapy for definition of GERD [22, 23]. The guidelines underscore the importance of objective testing in the definition of GERD.

The ACG guidelines also addressed the controversial clinical significance and causal relationship of atypical and extraesophageal manifestations, particularly those included as extraesophageal syndromes of proposed association in Montreal classification, because the association is largely based on weak evidence such as retrospective case-control studies.

The ACG guidelines commended the use of endoscopy as a specific tool of defining GERD through endoscopic detection of reflux esophagitis by Los Angeles classification. Endoscopy with biopsy is essential for the confirmation of intestinal metaplasia for Barrett's esophagus. Ambulatory reflux monitoring (pH or impedance-pH) helps define GERD by quantitative evaluation of the esophageal exposure to gastric refluxate and determination of chronological association between reflux events and symptom episodes [24–32].

Defining GERD in ASIA: Limitation of Montreal Classification and Other Western Definitions

Symptomatology

There is considerable heterogeneity in the prevalence and spectrum of GERD, peptic ulcer, and gastric cancer, making universal strategy for defining GERD very difficult in Asia [33]. Overlapping of GERD and functional gastrointestinal disorders is common, causing difficulty in distinguishing these conditions clinically [34–39]. GERD symptoms are still poorly recognized and undertreated in many Asian countries [33, 40].

Although the Montreal classification reported a high level of agreement on the meaning of heartburn, the definition and the specificity of these symptoms have been evaluated primarily in Caucasian populations, and there is a lack of data in Asia-Pacific region. While the typical reflux symptoms such as heartburn and acid regurgitation are increasingly comprehensible to Asian patients, the interpretation of these symptoms is generally poor in Asians. [41]. There is no equivalent term for "heartburn" in Asian languages, and the symptom of heartburn has different meanings in different Asian ethnic groups. These classical GERD symptoms are derived largely based on studies in Western populations and are generally poorly understood and inadequately validated in Asians.

Different frequency criteria of GERD symptoms have been used for defining GERD, with a frequency ranging from once a week to even once a year. There is still a lack of standardized definition in Asia. Besides typical symptoms, patients may also present with other symptoms such as chest pain, belching, nausea, dysphagia, early satiety, and epigastric pain, with or without typical reflux symptoms. Non-cardiac chest pain is commonly reported as a presenting feature of GERD in Asian patients [3, 42]. However, it has not been adequately recognized in the daily clinical practice. The reflux chest pain syndrome in Montreal classification helps highlight a distinct group of GERD patients who have chest pain as the presenting symptom.

In the Montreal classification, GERD is defined using symptom/frequency criteria. However, defining GERD based on frequency criteria may not be straightforward because reflux symptoms may not occur in a regular weekly manner. In real-life clinical practice, GERD is often defined by the presence of troublesome symptoms and quality of life impairment, regardless of the frequency. However, it has been observed that GERD patients identified by using these two different definitions do not overlap significantly. Further studies are needed to define the relative merit of frequency criteria and quality of life impairment for definition of GERD [43].

The association between GERD and extraesophageal syndromes has been conflicting in Asians. The value of anti-reflux treatment in the management of extraesophageal syndromes in Asian patients is also controversial. Although there are Asian studies that suggest significant association between typical reflux symptoms and chronic laryngitis, hoarseness, and asthma, GERD is rarely the sole cause of chronic cough, chronic laryngitis, or asthma in patients with no typical reflux symptoms or esophagitis [44–48]. This entity is highly controversial, with the lack of objective evidence by clinical trials and investigations. Furthermore, the low prevalence of GERD in Asia leads to low pretest probability and positive predictive value of diagnostic tests for GERD in patients with suspected extraesophageal syndromes.

On the other hand, sleep disturbance is commonly reported as a troublesome symptom in Asian GERD patients, but it has been largely neglected as a parameter for monitoring of treatment response in daily clinical practice.

In the Western population, symptomatic response to empirical trial of PPI therapy has long been used for diagnosis of GERD in patients with typical symptoms. However, the positive predictive value of PPI test is significantly associated with the prevalence of GERD relative to the other acid peptic disorders in the respective population. Owing to the relatively low prevalence of GERD and preponderance of peptic ulcer diseases in Asia, the pretest probability of PPI test may be substantially lower in Asian population. The validity of PPI trial for defining GERD needs to be defined in individual populations because of the heterogeneity in prevalence of GERD [49].

Role of Endoscopy and Other Reflux Investigations

The diagnostic yield of endoscopy for reflux syndrome with esophageal injury is low in the Asian population. Although reflux esophagitis serves as a specific and objective criterion for defining GERD, it is found in less than 50% of Asian patients with typical reflux symptoms and in less than 10% in those with reflux chest pain syndrome. The Los Angeles classification, the best validated classification system for evaluating erosive esophagitis, is underutilized by Asian endoscopists. Other less validated systems such as Savary Miller grading system are still commonly in use. The use of less accurate classification system leads to under- or overdiagnosis of esophagitis. Severe complications such as peptic stricture, Barrett's esophagus, and esophageal adenocarcinoma are rare, and the risk factors are not clearly defined. It has been reported that up to 40% of Barrett's esophagus in Chinese are asymptomatic [50].

Despite the low prevalence of GERD complications, endoscopy plays an important role in defining GERD in Asia. Endoscopy helps exclude the possibility of peptic ulcer disease and gastric cancer, which are highly prevalent and may mimic the symptoms of GERD. Prompt endoscopy in patients with alarm symptoms results in a significant yield of major upper gastrointestinal pathology such as cancer and peptic ulcer. There is no data on the direct comparison between the strategies of empirical PPI and prompt endoscopy as the most appropriate initial approach to GERD patients in Asia. However, it has been reported that 18% of *H. pylori*-related peptic ulcers were misdiagnosed as GERD based on symptoms alone [51]. The empirical use of PPI may also heal peptic ulcer and even early gastric cancer. The accuracy of *H. pylori* test will also be undermined by prior use of PPI. It is therefore advisable to arrange endoscopy before empirical PPI is contemplated. In areas where endoscopy is not readily accessible, other non-endoscopy modalities of *H. pylori* testing should be considered prior to empirical PPI trial in new patients presenting with GERD symptoms in regions with a high prevalence of gastric cancer or peptic ulcer disease [52].

It is important to note that peculiar endoscopic definition of esophageal injury related to GERD in some Asian countries. Image-enhanced endoscopic diagnosis of GERD is popular in Japan and Korea. The concept of "minimal change" esophagitis, which is defined as the white turbid discoloration and blurring of Z line, has been proposed as early sign of esophageal injury. It has been suggested that nonerosive reflux disease (NERD) should be further classified as "normal" and "minimal change," but whether these two entities are different in clinical characteristics and response to PPI treatment is still a subject of dispute [19, 53–57]. In Japan, the gastroesophageal junction is anatomically defined by the distal limit of the lower esophageal palisade vessels, in contrast to the conventionally designated proximal limit of gastric rugal folds. Because the distal limit of lower esophageal palisade vessels generally extends distally to the proximal gastric rugal folds, there is a prevailing concept of ultrashort segment Barrett's esophagus in the Japanese definition of the Barrett's esophagus. As a result, the prevalence estimates of columnar-lined esophagus (CLE) or Barrett's esophagus are substantially higher using the Japanese criteria. The validity and clinical relevance of the Japanese criteria have been questioned because intestinal metaplasia is rarely found in the Barrett's esophagus defined by these criteria [58]. There is no evidence that suggests these criteria are more predictive or better correlated with severe GERD or complications such as adenocarcinoma. The entity of endoscopically suspected esophageal metaplasia (ESEM) proposed in the Montreal classification has also been considered to introduce confusion and risk of overdiagnosis in Asians. Therefore, it is not recommended for daily clinical use in the Asian setting.

Although ambulatory reflux testing may help compensate for the poor diagnostic accuracy of symptomatology, it is not widely available in Asia. Most ambulatory reflux monitoring tests are done in major referral centers. Furthermore, there is still a lack of well-validated data on normal values in most Asian populations [59].

References

1. Kahrilas PJ, Shaheen NJ, Vaezi MF. American gastroenterological association institute technical review on the management of gastroesophageal reflux disease. Gastroenterology. 2008 Oct;135(4):1392–413.
2. Goh KL. Gastroesophageal reflux disease in Asia: a historical perspective and present challenges. J Gastroenterol Hepatol. 2011 Jan;26(Suppl 1):2–10.
3. Ho KY, Ng WL, Kang JY, Yeoh KG. Gastroesophageal reflux disease is a common cause of noncardiac chest pain in a country with a low prevalence of reflux esophagitis. Dig Dis Sci. 1998;43(9):1991–7.
4. Lim SL, Goh WT, Lee JM, Ng TP, Ho KY. Changing prevalence of gastroesophageal reflux with changing time: longitudinal study in an Asian population. J Gastroenterol Hepatol. 2005;20(7):995–1001.

5. Ho KY, Chan YH, Kang JY. Increasing trend of reflux esophagitis and decreasing trend of helicobacter pylori infection in patients from a multiethnic Asian country. Am J Gastroenterol. 2005;100(9):1923–8.

6. El-Serag HB, Sweet S, Winchester CC, Dent J. Update on the epidemiology of gastro-oesophageal reflux disease: a systematic review. Gut. 2014;63(6):871–80.

7. Goh KL. Obesity and increasing gastroesophageal reflux disease in Asia. J Gastroenterol Hepatol. 2007;22(10):1557–8.

8. Ho KY. Gastroesophageal reflux disease in Asia: a condition in evolution. J Gastroenterol Hepatol. 2008;23(5):716–22.

9. Wu JC. Gastroesophageal reflux disease: an Asian perspective. J Gastroenterol Hepatol. 2008;23(12):1785–93.

10. Fass R. Distinct phenotypic presentations of gastroesophageal reflux disease: a new view of the natural history. Dig Dis. 2004;22(2):100–7.

11. Wu JC, Cheung CM, Wong VW, Sung JJ. Distinct clinical characteristics between patients with nonerosive reflux disease and those with reflux esophagitis. Clin Gastroenterol Hepatol. 2007;5(6):690–5.

12. El-Serag HB. Epidemiology of non-erosive reflux disease. Digestion. 2008;78(Suppl 1):6–10.

13. Fass R. Non-erosive reflux disease (NERD) and erosive esophagitis–a spectrum of disease or special entities? Z Gastroenterol. 2007;45(11):1156–63.

14. Vakil N, van Zanten SV, Kahrilas P, Dent J, Jones R. The Montreal definition and classification of gastroesophageal reflux disease: a global evidence-based consensus. Am J Gastroenterol. 2006;101(8):1900–20.

15. Lundell LR, Dent J, Bennett JR, Blum AL, Armstrong D, Galmiche JP, et al. Endoscopic assessment of oesophagitis: clinical and functional correlates and further validation of the Los Angeles classification. Gut. 1999;45(2):172–80.

16. Sharma P, Wani S, Bansal A, Hall S, Puli S, Mathur S, et al. A feasibility trial of narrow band imaging endoscopy in patients with gastroesophageal reflux disease. Gastroenterology. 2007;133(2):454–64.

17. Lee YC, Lin JT, Chiu HM, Liao WC, Chen CC, Tu CH, et al. Intraobserver and interobserver consistency for grading esophagitis with narrow-band imaging. Gastrointest Endosc. 2007;66(2):230–6.

18. Gawron AJ, Hirano I. Advances in diagnostic testing for gastroesophageal reflux disease. World J Gastroenterol. 2010;16(30):3750–6.

19. Falk GW. Is conventional endoscopic identification of non-erosive reflux disease adequate? Digestion. 2008;78(Suppl 1):17–23.

20. Dent J. Endoscopic grading of reflux oesophagitis: the past, present and future. Best Pract Res Clin Gastroenterol. 2008;22(4):585–99.

21. Dent J, Becher A, Sung J, Zou D, Agreus L, Bazzoli F. Systematic review: patterns of reflux-induced symptoms and esophageal endoscopic findings in large-scale surveys. Clin Gastroenterol Hepatol. 2012;10(8):863–73.

22. Katz PO, Gerson LB, Vela MF. Guidelines for the diagnosis and management of gastroesophageal reflux disease. Am J Gastroenterol. 2013;108(3):308–28.

23. Numans ME, Lau J, de Wit NJ, Bonis PA. Short-term treatment with proton-pump inhibitors as a test for gastroesophageal reflux disease: a meta-analysis of diagnostic test characteristics. Ann Intern Med. 2004;140(7):518–27.

24. Kahrilas PJ, Hughes N, Howden CW. Response of unexplained chest pain to proton pump inhibitor treatment in patients with and without objective evidence of gastro-oesophageal reflux disease. Gut. 2011;60(11):1473–8.

25. Cremonini F, Wise J, Moayyedi P, Talley NJ. Diagnostic and therapeutic use of proton pump inhibitors in non-cardiac chest pain: a metaanalysis. Am J Gastroenterol. 2005;100(6):1226–32.

26. Dellon ES, Gonsalves N, Hirano I, Furuta GT, Liacouras CA, Katzka DA. ACG clinical guideline: evidenced based approach to the diagnosis and management of esophageal eosinophilia and eosinophilic esophagitis (EoE). Am J Gastroenterol. 2013;108(5):679–92.

27. Sperry SL, Shaheen NJ, Dellon ES. Toward uniformity in the diagnosis of eosinophilic esophagitis (EoE): the effect of guidelines on variability of diagnostic criteria for EoE. Am J Gastroenterol. 2011;106(5):824–32.

28. Hirano I, Richter JE. ACG practice guidelines: esophageal reflux testing. Am J Gastroenterol. 2007;102(3):668–85.

29. Hirano I, Zhang Q, Pandolfino JE, Kahrilas PJ. Four-day Bravo pH capsule monitoring with and without proton pump inhibitor therapy. Clin Gastroenterol Hepatol. 2005;3(11):1083–8.

30. Sifrim D, Castell D, Dent J, Kahrilas PJ. Gastro-oesophageal reflux monitoring: review and consensus report on detection and definitions of acid, non-acid, and gas reflux. Gut. 2004;53(7):1024–31.

31. Sinn DH, Kim BJ, Son HJ, Kim JJ, Rhee JC, Rhee PL. Pathological bolus exposure may define gastro-esophageal reflux better than pathological acid exposure in patients with globus. Hepato-Gastroenterology. 2012;59(114):317–20.

32. Connor J, Richter J. Increasing yield also increases false positives and best serves to exclude GERD. Am J Gastroenterol. 2006;101(3):460–3.

33. Ho KY, Kang JY, Seow A. Prevalence of gastrointestinal symptoms in a multiracial Asian population, with particular reference to reflux-type symptoms. Am J Gastroenterol. 1998;93(10):1816–22.

34. Gerson LB, Kahrilas PJ, Fass R. Insights into gastroesophageal reflux disease-associated dyspeptic symptoms. Clin Gastroenterol Hepatol. 2011;9(10):824–33.

35. Choi JY, Jung HK, Song EM, Shim KN, Jung SA. Determinants of symptoms in gastroesophageal reflux disease: nonerosive reflux disease, symptomatic, and silent erosive reflux disease. Eur J Gastroenterol Hepatol. 2013;25(7):764–71.

36. Ghoshal UC, Singh R, Chang FY, Hou X, Wong BC, Kachintorn U. Epidemiology of uninvestigated and functional dyspepsia in Asia: facts and fiction. J Neurogastroenterol Motil. 2011;17(3):235–44.

37. Hongo M. Epidemiology of FGID symptoms in Japanese general population with reference to life style. J Gastroenterol Hepatol. 2011;26(Suppl 3):19–22.

38. Park H. Functional gastrointestinal disorders and overlap syndrome in Korea. J Gastroenterol Hepatol. 2011;26(Suppl 3):12–4.

39. Kaji M, Fujiwara Y, Shiba M, Kohata Y, Yamagami H, Tanigawa T, et al. Prevalence of overlaps between GERD, FD and IBS and impact on health-related quality of life. J Gastroenterol Hepatol. 2010;25(6):1151–6.

40. Bor S, Mandiracioglu A, Kitapcioglu G, Caymaz-Bor C, Gilbert RJ. Gastroesophageal reflux disease in a low-income region in Turkey. Am J Gastroenterol. 2005;100(4):759–65.

41. Spechler SJ, Jain SK, Tendler DA, Parker RA. Racial differences in the frequency of symptoms and complications of gastro-oesophageal reflux disease. Aliment Pharmacol Ther. 2002;16(10):1795–800.

42. Mohd H, Qua CS, Wong CH, Azman W, Goh KL. Non-cardiac chest pain: prevalence of reflux disease and response to acid suppression in an Asian population. J Gastroenterol Hepatol. 2009;24(2):288–93.

43. Wang R, Zou D, Ma X, Zhao Y, Yan X, Yan H, et al. Impact of gastroesophageal reflux disease on daily life: the systematic investigation of gastrointestinal diseases in China (SILC) epidemiological study. Health Qual Life Outcomes. 2010;8:128.

44. Qua CS, Wong CH, Gopala K, Goh KL. Gastro-oesophageal reflux disease in chronic laryngitis: prevalence and response to acid-suppressive therapy. Aliment Pharmacol Ther. 2007;25(3):287–95.

45. Tsai MC, Lin HL, Lin CC, Lin HC, Chen YH, Pfeiffer S, et al. Increased risk of concurrent asthma among patients with gastroesophageal reflux disease: a nationwide population-based study. Eur J Gastroenterol Hepatol. 2010;22(10):1169–73.

46. Amarasiri LD, Pathmeswaran A, de Silva HJ, Ranasinha CD. Prevalence of gastro-oesophageal reflux disease symptoms and reflux-associated respiratory symptoms in asthma. BMC Pulm Med. 2010;10:49.

47. Jaimchariyatam N, Wongtim S, Udompanich V, Sittipunt C, Kawkitinarong K, Chaiyakul S, et al. Prevalence of gastroesophageal reflux in Thai asthmatic patients. J Med Assoc Thail. 2011;94(6):671–8.

48. Lam P, Wei WI, Hui Y, Ho WK. Prevalence of pH-documented laryngopharyngeal reflux in Chinese patients with clinically suspected reflux laryngitis. Am J Otolaryngol. 2006;27(3):186–9.

49. Cho YK, Choi MG, Lim CH, Nam KW, Chang JH, Park JM, et al. Diagnostic value of the PPI test for detection of GERD in Korean patients and factors associated with PPI responsiveness. Scand J Gastroenterol. 2010;45(5):533–9.

50. Peng S, Cui Y, Xiao YL, Xiong LS, Hu PJ, Li CJ, et al. Prevalence of erosive esophagitis and Barrett's esophagus in the adult Chinese population. Endoscopy. 2009;41(12):1011–7.

51. Wu JC, Chan FK, Ching JY, Leung WK, Lee YT, Sung JJ. Empirical treatment based on "typical" reflux symptoms is inappropriate in a population with a high prevalence of helicobacter pylori infection. Gastrointest Endosc. 2002;55(4):461–5.

52. Fock KM, Talley NJ, Fass R, Goh KL, Katelaris P, Hunt R, et al. Asia-Pacific consensus on the management of gastroesophageal reflux disease: update. J Gastroenterol Hepatol. 2008;23(1):8–22.

53. Lee JH, Kim N, Chung IK, Jo YJ, Seo GS, Kim SW, et al. Clinical significance of minimal change lesions of the esophagus in a healthy Korean population: a nationwide multi-center prospective study. J Gastroenterol Hepatol. 2008;23(7 Pt 1):1153–7.

54. Lei WY, Liu TT, Yi CH, Chen CL. Disease characteristics in non-erosive reflux disease with and without endoscopically minimal change esophagitis: are they different? Digestion. 2012;85(1):27–32.

55. Kim JH, Park H, Lee YC. Is minimal change esophagitis really part of the spectrum of endoscopic findings of gastroesophageal reflux disease? A prospective, multicenter study. Endoscopy. 2011;43(3):190–5.

56. Miwa H, Yokoyama T, Hori K, Sakagami T, Oshima T, Tomita T, et al. Interobserver agreement in endoscopic evaluation of reflux esophagitis using a modified Los Angeles classification incorporating grades N and M: a validation study in a cohort of Japanese endoscopists. Dis Esophagus. 2008;21(4):355–63.

57. Kiesslich R, Kanzler S, Vieth M, Moehler M, Neidig J, Thanka Nadar BJ, et al. Minimal change esophagitis: prospective comparison of endoscopic and histological markers between patients with non-erosive reflux disease and normal controls using magnifying endoscopy. Dig Dis. 2004;22(2):221–7.

58. Ogiya K, Kawano T, Ito E, Nakajima Y, Kawada K, Nishikage T, et al. Lower esophageal palisade vessels and the definition of Barrett's esophagus. Dis Esophagus. 2008;21(7):645–9.

59. Xiao YL, Lin JK, Cheung TK, Wong NY, Yang L, Hung IF, et al. Normal values of 24-hour combined esophageal multichannel intraluminal impedance and pH monitoring in the Chinese population. Digestion. 2009;79(2):109–14.

Epidemiology of Gastroesophageal Reflux in Asia

Shobna Bhatia, Deepak Kumar Gupta, and Prashanth Vennalaganti

Abstract

Gastroesophageal reflux disease (GERD) is the most common gastrointestinal complaint seen across the world. It has often been perceived as Western disease due to its high prevalence of around 10–20%. In Asia, limited data showed that the prevalence was 2.5–6.7% and that most patients had mild disease. However, within the last decade, research in GERD showed that the prevalence of weekly heartburn ranges from 8 to 20%, which is higher than previous estimates; however, erosive esophagitis was seen in less than 20% of patients. This increase in prevalence could be due to the changing dynamics mainly due to interaction of environmental, genetic, and recent socioeconomical development in Asia. The diversity in ethnic populations in Asia leads to problem in evaluation of the prevalence of gastroesophageal disease mainly due to the cultural, social, and language differences. The aim of this chapter is to review the epidemiological studies of gastroesophageal disease, including those of erosive esophagitis and Barrett's esophagus in Asia, and provide an understanding of the regional variation and the changes seen over the last decade.

Keywords

Heartburn • Sour regurgitation • Natural history • Nonerosive reflux disease • Erosive esophagitis

S. Bhatia (✉)
Gastroenterology, KEM Hospital, Mumbai, Maharashtra, India
e-mail: shobna.bhatia@gmail.com

D.K. Gupta
Deparment of Gastroenterology, Seth GS Medical College and KEM Hospital, Acharya Donde Marg, Parel, Mumbai, India, 400012

P. Vennalaganti
Department of Gastroenterology and Hepatology, University of Kansas School of Medicine, Kansas City, KS, USA

© Springer India 2018
P. Sharma et al. (eds.), *The Rise of Acid Reflux in Asia*,
DOI 10.1007/978-81-322-0846-4_2

Introduction

Gastroesophageal reflux disease (GERD) is one of the most commonly encountered gastrointestinal disease in the world. GERD is a spectrum of disease which includes symptoms like heartburn or regurgitation to complications like erosive esophagitis, Barrett's esophagus, and related neoplasia. GERD is a condition which develops when the reflux of the stomach contents causes troublesome symptoms and/or complication, as per Montreal definition of GERD [1]. GERD affects 10–20% of the adult population in the USA and Europe [1]. These figures are likely an underestimate of its true prevalence, since many patients self-medicate and/or do not seek medical advice. GERD is often perceived as a Western disease due to limited literature among the Asian population. The reported population prevalence of GERD in Eastern Asia ranges from 2.5 to 6.7% [2].

In the last decade, the Asia-Pacific region has carried out active research in GERD. Increasing incidence of GERD has been noted among various Asian countries in the last 10 years. The aim of this chapter, therefore, is to review the epidemiologic studies of GERD in Asia, including those of erosive esophagitis, and to provide a realistic understanding of the change of prevalence of GERD over time.

History of GERD in Asia

The regions of Asia include: Eastern (China, Japan, Korea, and Taiwan), Southeastern (Malaysia, Singapore, and Thailand), South Central (India, Iran, Pakistan, and Bangladesh) and Western (Israel and Turkey). The first report in the published English medical literature on GERD was by Kang and colleagues in 1993 [2]. Prior to that, in the late 1970s, two reports from Taiwan mentioned the presence of esophagitis among patients who had undergone gastroscopy [3, 4]. In 2005, Dent and colleagues estimated that the prevalence of GERD was 10–20% in Western countries and approximately 5% in Asia, in a systematic review of studies that defined GERD as symptoms of heartburn and/or regurgitation occurring on at least 1 day per week [1]. Similarly, in another systematic review, the prevalence of GERD in Asia was estimated to range between 2.5 and 6.7% [5]. However, recently many studies from Asia have shown an increasing trend in the prevalence of GERD. There are substantial differences in GERD prevalence among Asian regions. The prevalence is highest in West Asia (12.5–27.6%), less so in Central Asia (7.6–19.4%), and lowest in East Asia (2.5–9.4%) [7].

Measuring the Burden of GERD

The exact burden of GERD is difficult to measure, as endoscopy only measures erosive esophagitis. The true prevalence of GERD in the community with questionnaire or direct questioning will also provide vital information in estimating the prevalence, as a large number of people who suffer from GERD do not visit a physician for this complaint. There are also some language and cultural differences in symptom interpretation such as the lack of the exact word for heartburn in some Asian languages, making it difficult to accurately estimate the prevalence of GERD in these populations. For example, in Korean, Malay, and Chinese, there is no direct word describing the symptom, and a survey in the USA revealed that only 13.2% of East Asian patients understood the term [6]. There are only a few population-based studies from Asia that have used the Montreal definition or definitions that are close to it.

Prevalence of GERD: Symptom-Based Studies

Eastern Asia (China, Japan, Korea, and Taiwan)

In Eastern Asia, various large-scale population studies have been conducted. The prevalence of GERD was estimated between 6.6 and 20.7% among various populations. In a cross-sectional study by Fukujima et al., the prevalence of GERD was estimated at 6.6% among patients who visited physicians for a routine physical exam. In another survey of 1076 patients who presented with epigastric symptoms between April and August 2007 at 55 institutions in Japan, the prevalence of GERD was estimated at 15.6%, and in another study of 160,973 adults who presented for screening of gastric carcinoma and reported abdominal pain, the prevalence of GERD was between 15.8 and 20.7% [7–9].

The prevalence of GERD in China is estimated to be between 1.7 and 7.3%. The largest population-based study among 16,091 subjects by He et al., based on self-reported questionnaire, estimated the prevalence of GERD as 3.1%, varying between 1.7 and 5.1% in different regions [10]. Li et al., in a survey of more than 15, 000 outpatients attending hospitals in Zhejiang province, China, recorded a prevalence of 7.3% [11]. The prevalence of GERD in Shanghai (Weng et al.) and South China (Chen et al.) based on population-based studies was approximately 6.2% [12–14]. The prevalence was even lower in Hong Kong, where the prevalence rates of GERD, as estimated by telephonic interviews, were between 0.25 and 4.8% [15, 16].

The prevalence of GERD in South Korea was estimated to be similar to the Western countries at 7.1%, based on telephone interviews among the general population. Based on another population-based study [17] and telephone survey [18] in Korea, its prevalence was estimated at 3.5 and 8.5%, respectively. In Taiwan, using a modified GERD questionnaire, Lu et al. recorded prevalence of 6.6% as once-weekly symptoms [19]. A recent review of changing GERD trends showed that prevalence of symptom-based GERD in Eastern Asia was 5.2–8.5% [4–9, 20, 21] from 2005 to 2010, whereas it was 2.5–4.8% [11, 13, 14] before 2005. However, it has stricter criteria for GERD definition for inclusion of the studies.

Southeastern Asia (Malaysia, Singapore, and Thailand)

In Singapore, Ho et al. showed the highest prevalence among Indians (7.5%) and Malays (3%) [22]. In another study that surveyed the same cohort in 1994 and in 1999, the prevalence of GERD was 5.5% ± 1.5% initially, but increased to

10.5% ± 2.0% after 5 years [23]. In Malaysia, Rajendra and Alahuddin in 2004 showed symptomatic prevalence of 9.7% based on patients having monthly symptoms [24]. In Thailand, a study by the Thai motility club (using questionnaire) reported a 7.4% prevalence of GERD in community (unpublished data) (esophagitis 4–6%) [26].

South Central Asia (India, Iran, Pakistan, and Bangladesh)

Most studies in South Central Asia were conducted in Iran. The prevalence of GERD in Iran was 6.3–18.3% from 2005 to 2010, and higher than in Eastern Asia [25–27]. The prevalence of GERD in Bangladesh ranged from 5.3 to 19.4% [28, 29]. Jafri et al. reported a prevalence of 24% in Pakistan in 2005 [30]. The prevalence of GERD in India was estimated at 7.6% in a large prospective multicenter study involving 12 centers and 3224 subjects in 2011 [31]. The prevalence of GERD in other questionnaire-based cross-sectional studies ranged between 10.6 and 18.7% [32–34].

West Asia (Israel and Turkey)

The prevalence of GERD in West Asia was found to be the highest in all of Asia. The prevalence was found to be 20–27.6% in Turkey [35–37]. However, the symptom profile of the Turkish people was said to differ considerably; they have a relatively lower occurrence of heartburn and a higher incidence of regurgitation and dyspepsia. In Israel, Moshkowitz et al. reported prevalence of 12.5% of GERD symptoms [38]. Another population-based study in 2007 also reported a high prevalence of GERD symptoms, including retrosternal burning in 6.5%, retrosternal pain in 5.2%, acid taste in the mouth in 10.4%, and reflux of gastric contents in 7.9% of subjects [39]. Prevalence of GERD in population-based studies is higher in Central and West Asia than in East Asia [38].

Selected studies highlighting the prevalence of reflux symptoms in Asia after year 2000

Study, year [reference]	Country	Method	Sample size	Prevalence of reflux symptoms (%) Daily/at least weekly/at least monthly/at least yearly
Eastern Asia				
Stanghellini 1999 [21]	Japan (part of international study	*Digest* Random house-to-house recruitment	500	Prevalence of 9.8% for heartburn and of 3.6% for regurgitation
Fujiwara et al. 2005 [7]	Kansai, Japan	Questionnaire	6035 (clinic based)	Prevalence of 12.8% (> 2 per month)
He et al. 2010 [10]	China	Self-reported questionnaires	16,091	At least weekly, 5.2%; at least twice a week, 3.1% (2.4% in urban and 3.8% in rural area)

(continued)

Study, year [reference]	Country	Method	Sample size	Prevalence of reflux symptoms (%) Daily/at least weekly/at least monthly/at least yearly
Pan et al. 2000 [40]	China	Assisted self-completed questionnaire (*GERQ*)	4992	HB 2.5/HB 3.1/HB 7.0
Hu et al. 2002	China	Telephone interview (bowel symptom questionnaire)	2640	4.8
Wong et al. 2003 [16]	China	Telephone interview (*GERQ*)	3605	2.5/8.9/29.8
Cho et al. 2005 [17]	Korea	Face-to-face interview (*GERQ*)	1902	GERD 3.5/HB 4.7/AR 4.4 2.0/AR 2.0
Fujiwara et al. 2005 [7]	Japan	Face-to-face interview	6035	2.1/6.6/19.4/44.1
Western & Southern Asia				
Bor et al. 2005 [35]	Turkey	Face-to-face interview (*GERQ*)	630	4.9/GERD 20/HB GERD 37.6/HB 10/AR 15.6, 15.9/AR 32.7 9, AR 32.7
Nouraie et al. 2007	Iran	Face-to-face interview	2561	GERD 21.2/HB 12.2/AR 16.8
Pourshams et al. 2007	Iran	Face-to-face interview	1000	12.3
Sperber et al. 2007 [39]	Israel	Telephone interview (*RDQ*)	1221	0.3/9.3
Bhatia et al. 2011 [85]	India	Questionnaire	3224	Heartburn 2.7/3.2/12.7 Regurgitation 2.0/2.3/9.2

GERQ gastroesophageal reflux questionnaire, *HB* heartburn, *AR* acid regurgitation, *RDQ* reflux disease questionnaire

Prevalence of Esophagitis

Most endoscopy-based studies were conducted on subjects with upper gastrointestinal symptoms in tertiary care hospitals.

Eastern Asia (China, Japan, Korea, and Taiwan)

Using the Los Angeles classification, the prevalence was estimated between 6.6 and 15.0% [41–45] from nine studies between 2000 and 2005 and 4.3–15.7% [46–49] after 2005. Several studies were conducted in retrospective manner and may have under- or overestimated the exact prevalence of endoscopic reflux esophagitis. SILC study, [50] a population-based endoscopy study conducted in China, showed symptomatic GERD to be more prevalent among patients who agreed to endoscopy (4.7% vs. 1.7%). Among patients who underwent endoscopy, the prevalence of erosive esophagitis was 6.4% (Los Angeles grade A 4.1%, grade B 2.1%, grade C 0.2%, and grade D 0%, respectively). Erosive esophagitis was also more prevalent among patients with symptomatic GERD (12.5% vs. 6.1%).

Southeastern Asia (Malaysia, Singapore, and Thailand)

In Malaysia, the prevalence of erosive esophagitis was estimated at 13.4% among 1000 patients with upper abdominal discomfort [51]. Similarly, Rajendra et al. showed prevalence of erosive esophagitis as 6.1% in 1985 patients with abdominal discomfort or reflux [52]. In Singapore, several studies showed prevalence of reflux esophagitis between 5 and 6.9% [53, 52].

Western Asia (Israel and Turkey)

In Saudi Arabia, Al-Humayed et al. reported a prevalence of 15% in 1607 patients who underwent endoscopy for evaluation of dyspepsia [54]. A retrospective analysis of 18,766 endoscopies by Yilmaz et al. in Turkey between 1996 and 2001 reported prevalence of erosive esophagitis as 12.8% [54].

Prevalence of Extra-Esophageal Syndromes

Extra-esophageal syndromes include respiratory symptoms, such as chronic cough, asthma, or laryngitis, dental erosions, noncardiac chest pain (NCCP), and sleep disturbance [55]. In a study by Shimizu et al. [56], the proportion of endoscopic reflux esophagitis in patients with asthma was higher than in controls (39.3% vs. 0.6%). The proportion of sleep dysfunction was 52.5–56.6% among the patients with GERD [57–59]. In tertiary hospitals in China, dental erosions were found in 64.5% among patients with frequent reflux symptoms (three to five times per week), 44.4% among subjects with occasional symptoms (one to two times per week), and 36.7% among controls ($p < 0.05$) [60]. The prevalence of GERD among patients with NCCP was 66.7% and 20%, respectively, in Malaysia [61] and Turkey [35].

Selected Studies Highlighting the Prevalence of Erosive Esophagitis in Asia

Study, year [reference]	Country	Target population	Sample size	Prevalence of esophagitis (%)
Southern Asia				
Khuroo et al., 1989	India	Patients with dyspepsia	239	5.60
Nasseri-Moghaddam et al., 2003	Iran	Patients with dyspepsia referred for upper endoscopy	269	76.90
Southeastern Asia				
Kang et al., 1993 [2]	Singapore	Patients with upper GI symptoms (inpatients and outpatients)	11,943	4.50

(continued)

Study, year [reference]	Country	Target population	Sample size	Prevalence of esophagitis (%)
Rosaida et al., 2004 [51]	Malaysia	Patients with upper abdominal discomfort	1000	13.40
Eastern Asia				
Yeh et al., 1997 [62]	Taiwan	Patients with upper GI symptoms (heartburn, regurgitation, epigastric pain, and GI bleeding)	464	14.50
Yeom et al., 1999	Korea	Patients with GI tract symptoms	1010	5.30
Furukawa et al., 1999 [63]	Japan	Patients requiring routine physical examinations	6010	16.30
Inamori et al., 2003 [64]	Japan	First time endoscopy in patients with heartburn, dyspepsia, noncardiac chest pain	392	13.80
Western Asia Toruner et al., 2004	Turkey	Patients with dyspepsia referred for upper endoscopy	395	15.40

Prevalence of Barrett's Esophagus

Barrett's esophagus is histologically confirmed by specialized intestinal metaplasia in biopsies from a columnar-lined distal esophagus. Epidemiologic studies have consistently reported that the prevalence of Barrett's esophagus-associated adenocarcinoma is very rare in Asia [65, 66]. Among 19,812 consecutive Chinese patients undergoing upper endoscopy for routine health examination between June 2003 and December 2006, Barrett's esophagus (BE) was confirmed only in 0.06% [45]. In another large Korean retrospective analysis of 70,103 patients undergoing upper endoscopy, 1% had suspected CLE. Of these patients, BE was histologically confirmed in 0.22% [67]. In the earliest study on Barrett's esophagus from Asia confirmed on histopathology, Yeh et al. reported a prevalence of 2% [65].

The prevalence of Barrett's esophagus was reported between 0.3 and 2% [62, 68–73] in tertiary hospitals from various regions of Asia. Recent large studies from Korea and Taiwan have yielded prevalence rates of 0.01 and 0.03% for LSBE and 0.14 and 2.4% for SSBE, respectively [45, 67]. In India, Amarapukar et al. showed prevalence of 2.6% [74]. It has been commented previously that Japanese studies report a higher prevalence of Barrett's owing to a different definition of the gastroesophageal junction [73].

Changing GERD Trends in Asia

The prevalence rates of both GERD symptoms and erosive esophagitis in a majority of recent reports have, in general, been higher than in earlier studies. This may be due to better diagnosis and recording of cases, but consistently higher rates from many centers in Asia are more likely to reflect a true increase in the prevalence of GERD.

A recent survey of 221 gastroenterologists, 205 primary care physicians, and 159 otolaryngologists across seven nations in Asia revealed that most (gastroenterologists, 90%; primary care physicians, 67%; otolaryngologists, 65%) perceive a rising occurrence of GERD [75]. Although there is a lack of longitudinal studies on the same source population to determine absolute change of GERD prevalence over time, recent reports from cross-sectional studies conducted across Asia indicate a general upward trend in the prevalence of GERD, [23, 43] with a rising proportion of patients presenting with reflux esophagitis [23, 43] and Barrett's esophagus or metaplasia [43, 75].

In a longitudinal five-year follow-up study looking at reflux symptoms, Lim et al. from Singapore reported a rise in the prevalence of reflux symptoms from 1.6 to 9.9% [23]. In another study from a small town in Western Japan over a 6-year period, 15.4% of GERD cases were identified as new cases [76]. More studies on changes in prevalence of reflux esophagitis with time have been carried out. Ho et al. from Singapore tracked the prevalence of esophagitis in their endoscopy records over a nine-year period and recorded an increase from 3.9 to 9.8% [53]. A study of 23,870 upper gastrointestinal endoscopies in a single Japanese center provides support for the Singapore results, showing the prevalence of reflux esophagitis increased from 0.8% in 1975–1977 to 2.3% in 1995–1997 [77].

Cross-sectional studies in Asia have also shown rising prevalence of GERD. In Korea, a study around 2005–2007 showed a GERD prevalence of 8.2% based on weekly symptoms of heartburn and/or acid regurgitation; this compares with the mere 3.5% based on the same criteria reported in a 2000–2001 study [17, 43]. Similarly, a 2003 study from South China estimated the prevalence of GERD based on weekly symptoms of heartburn and/or acid regurgitation at 6.2%, [12] in contrast to the modest 3.1% based on weekly heartburn reported by a study conducted in Beijing and Shanghai approximately a decade ago [78].

Erosive esophagitis prevalence has also shown a similar trend. The prevalence of endoscopic reflux esophagitis in Eastern Asia was 3.4–5.0% [77, 78] before 2000, and 6.6–15.0% [41–45] from 2000 to 2005. Japan witnessed an almost fivefold increase in the prevalence of esophagitis (latest figures are 13.8% of patients who underwent their first upper gastrointestinal endoscopy and 16.3% of patients on routine physical examinations) since the 1970s [63, 82].

Rising prevalence is also evident in Korea where the most recent (2004–2005) study reported finding reflux esophagitis in 18.8% of all dyspeptic patients undergoing EGD; [79] this is more than fivefold that reported a decade ago (3.4% during the period 1996–1998) [77] and is the highest esophagitis rate reported in Southeast and East Asia thus far.

On the heels of this rising trend are Malaysia and Taiwan, where esophagitis was seen in 13.4% (patients who underwent endoscopy) [51] and 14.5% (patients with upper gastrointestinal symptoms) [62]. The study, conducted at a single center in Malaysia, saw an almost fivefold increase within the decade encompassing the 1990s and early 2000s. On a smaller scale, the Philippines witnessed a twofold increase in esophagitis prevalence (6.3% vs. 2.9%, based on endoscopic diagnoses) within a span of approximately 10 years from 1992 [80]. However, despite the remarkable upsurge in prevalence, the esophagitis cases seen in the region remain largely mild; more than 80% of the cases in the above-mentioned Japanese and Malaysian studies were grade A type according to Los Angeles classification.

Why is GERD Increasing in Asia?

Most Asian patients have nonerosive GERD; erosive esophagitis is less commonly seen than in the Western population. Asians are known to be less predisposed to GERD than Caucasians due to their inherent smaller gastric parietal cell mass and lower acid output, low body mass index, lower obesity, lower consumption of alcohol, and probably also their traditional low-fat diet [81]. A high prevalence of *H. pylori* in Asia is also accounted as a reason for low GERD predisposition [53]. There is evidence to suggest that changing dynamics in various risk and protective factors contribute to both an increased incidence and severity of GERD in Asia. Despite these theories, the exact reason for the increasing trend in GERD in Asia is difficult to determine. This has been proposed as a result of interaction of environmental and genetic factors. The increase in prevalence occurring over a relatively short period of time (10–20 years) points to the predominant role of environmental factors. The growing affluence and socioeconomic development in Asia has resulted in consequent lifestyle changes. A change in diet and physical activity and an increase in BMI and obesity have often been thought to be putative. Also, life expectancy has now increased markedly, and a higher prevalence of GERD could also reflect the aging of the population.

Summary

There is evidence to suggest that changing dynamics in various risk and protective factors contribute to both an increased incidence and severity of GERD in Asia. It is therefore of utmost importance for both primary care physicians and specialists to increase vigilance for this emerging disease. General public awareness is required to facilitate early intervention for risk factors, more accurate diagnoses, and appropriate treatment. The development and validation of diagnostic questionnaires that are universally applicable in Asian countries of different ethnic and cultural origins are challenging tasks, but it is necessary to facilitate research into the epidemiology of GERD in Asia. Further studies are required to elucidate the clinical course of GERD and the time trend of its complications, such as Barrett's esophagus and adenocarcinoma of the esophagus. Differences may also be attributed to referral patterns, diagnostic practices, and physician recognition.

References

1. Dent J, El-Serag HB, Wallander MA, et al. Epidemiology of gastro-oesophageal reflux disease: a systematic review. Gut. 2005;54:710–7.
2. Kang JY, Tay HH, Yap I, Guan R, Lim KP, Math MV. Low frequency of endoscopic esophagitis in Asian patients. J Clin Gastroenterol. 1993;16:70–3.
3. Chen PC, Wu CS, Chang-Chien CS, Liaw YF. Comparison of Olympus GIF-P2 and GIF-K panendoscopy. Taiwan Yi Xue Hui Za Zhi. 1979;78:136–40. [Article in Chinese]
4. Wang TH, Lai MY, Lin RT, Wu CF, Chen DS, Wang CY, et al. Clinical experience with the upper gastrointestinal panendoscope GIF-P(2) (Olympus) (author's transl). Taiwan Yi Xue Hui Za Zhi. 1978;77:44–55.
5. Wong BC, Kinoshita Y. Systematic review on epidemiology of gastroesophageal reflux disease in Asia. Clin Gastroenterol Hepatol. 2006;4:398–407.
6. Agréus L, Svärdsudd K, Nyrén O, Tibblin G. Reproducibility and validity of a postal questionnaire. The abdominal symptom study. Scand J Prim Health Care. 1993;11:252–62.
7. Fujiwara Y, Higuchi K, Watanabe Y, Shiba M, Watanabe T, Tominaga K, et al. Prevalence of gastroesophageal reflux disease and gastroesophageal reflux disease symptoms in Japan. J Gastroenterol Hepatol. 2005;20:26–9.
8. Ohara S, Kawano T, Kusano M, Kouzu T. Survey on the prevalence of GERD and FD based on the Montreal definition and the Rome III criteria among patients presenting with epigastric symptoms in Japan. J Gastroenterol. 2011;46:603–11.
9. Yamagishi H, Koike T, Ohara S, Kobayashi S, Ariizumi K, Abe Y, et al. Prevalence of gastroesophageal reflux symptoms in a large unselected general population in Japan. World J Gastroenterol. 2008;14:1358–64.
10. He J, Ma X, Zhao Y, Wang R, Yan X, Yan H, et al. A population-based survey of the epidemiology of symptom-defined gastroesophageal reflux disease: the systematic investigation of gastrointestinal diseases in China. BMC Gastroenterol. 2010;10:94.
11. Li YM, Du J, Zhang H, Yu CH. Epidemiological investigation in outpatients with symptomatic gastroesophageal reflux from the Department of Medicine in Zhejiang Province, east China. J Gastroenterol Hepatol. 2008;23:283–9.
12. Chen M, Xiong L, Chen H, Xu A, He L, Hu P. Prevalence, risk factors and impact of gastroesophageal reflux disease symptoms: a population-based study in South China. Scand J Gastroenterol. 2005;40:759–67.
13. Ma XQ, Cao Y, Wang R, Yan X, Zhao Y, Zou D, et al. Prevalence of, and factors associated with, gastroesophageal reflux disease: a population-based study in shanghai. China Dis Esophagus. 2009;22:317–22.
14. Wang R, Yan X, Ma XQ, Cao Y, Wallander MA, Johansson S, et al. Burden of gastroesophageal reflux disease in shanghai. China Dig Liver Dis. 2009;41:110–5.
15. Cheung TK, Lam KF, Hu WH, Lam CL, Wong WM, Hui WM, et al. Positive association between gastro-oesophageal reflux disease and irritable bowel syndrome in a Chinese population. Aliment Pharmacol Ther. 2007;25:1099–104.
16. Wong WM, Lai KC, Lam KF, Hui WM, Hu WH, Lam CL, et al. Prevalence, clinical spectrum and health care utilization of gastro-oesophageal reflux disease in a Chinese population: a population-based study. Aliment Pharmacol Ther. 2003;18:595–604.
17. Cho YS, Choi MG, Jeong JJ, Chung WC, Lee IS, Kim SW, et al. Prevalence and clinical spectrum of gastroesophageal reflux: a population-based study in Asan-si. Korea Am J Gastroenterol. 2005;100:747–53.

18. Lee SY, Lee KJ, Kim SJ, Cho SW. Prevalence and risk factors for overlaps between gastroesophageal reflux disease, dyspepsia, and irritable bowel syndrome: a population-based study. Digestion. 2009;79:196–201.

19. Lu CL, Lang HC, Chang FY, Chen TJ, Chen CY, Luo JC, et al. Social and medical impact, sleep quality and the pharmaceutical costs of heartburn in Taiwan. Aliment Pharmacol Ther. 2005;22:739–47.

20. Ronkainen J, Agreus L. Epidemiology of reflux symptoms and GORD. Best Pract Res Clin Gastroenterol. 2013;27:325–37.

21. Stanghellini V. Relationship between upper gastrointestinal symptoms and lifestyle, psychosocial factors and comorbidity in the general population: results from the domestic/international gastroenterology surveillance study (DIGEST). Scand J Gastroenterol Suppl. 1999;231:29–37.

22. Ho KY, Kang JY, Seow A. Prevalence of gastrointestinal symptoms in a multiracial Asian population, with particular reference to reflux-type symptoms. Am J Gastroenterol. 1998;93:1816–22.

23. Lim SL, Goh WT, Lee JM, Ng TP, Ho KY; Community Medicine GI Study Group. Changing prevalence of gastroesophageal reflux with changing time: longitudinal study in an Asian population. J Gastroenterol Hepatol 2005;20:995–1001.

24. Rajendra S, Alahuddin S. Racial differences in the prevalence of heartburn. Aliment Pharmacol Ther. 2004;19:375–6.

25. Nasseri-Moghaddam S, Mofid A, Ghotbi MH, Razjouyan H, Nouraie M, Ramard AR, et al. Epidemiological study of gastro-oesophageal reflux disease: reflux in spouse as a risk factor. Aliment Pharmacol Ther. 2008;28:144–53.

26. Solhpour A, Pourhoseingholi MA, Soltani F, Zarghi A, Habibi M, Ghafarnejad F, et al. Gastroesophageal reflux symptoms and body mass index: no relation among the Iranian population. Indian J Gastroenterol. 2008;27:153–5.

27. Somi MH, Farhang S, Mirinezhad K, Jazayeri E, Nasseri-Moghaddam S, Moayeri S, et al. Prevalence and precipitating factors of gastroesophageal reflux disease in a young population of Tabriz. Northwest Iran Saudi Med J. 2006;27:1878–81.

28. Rokonuzzaman SM, Bhuian MR, Ali MH, Paul GK, Khan MR, Mamun AA. Epidemiological study of gastro-esophageal reflux disease in rural population. Mymensingh Med J. 2011;20:463–71.

29. Shaha M, Perveen I, Alamgir MJ, Masud MH, Rahman MH. Prevalence and risk factors for gastro-esophageal reflux disease in the north-eastern part of Bangladesh. Bangladesh Med Res Counc Bull. 2012;38:108–13.

30. Jafri N, Jafri W, Yakoob J, Islam M, Manzoor S, Jalil A, et al. Perception of gastroesophageal reflux disease in urban population in Pakistan. J Coll Physicians Surg Pak. 2005;15:532–4.

31. Bhatia SJ, Reddy DN, Ghoshal UC, Jayanthi V, Abraham P, Choudhuri G, et al. Epidemiology and symptom profile of gastroesophageal reflux in the Indian population: report of the Indian Society of Gastroenterology Task Force. Indian J Gastroenterol. 2011;30(3):118.

32. Shah SS, Bhatia SJ, Mistry FP. Epidemiology of dyspepsia in the general population in Mumbai. Indian J Gastroenterol. 2001;20:103–6.

33. Sharma PK, Ahuja V, Madan K, Gupta S, Raizada A, Sharma MP. Prevalence, severity, and risk factors of symptomatic gastroesophageal reflux disease among employees of a large hospital in northern India. Indian J Gastroenterol. 2011;30:128–34.

34. Kumar S, Sharma S, Norboo T, Dolma D, Norboo A, Stobdan T, et al. Population based study to assess prevalence and risk factors of gastroesophageal reflux disease in a high altitude area. Indian J Gastroenterol. 2011;30:135–43.

35. Bor S, Mandiracioglu A, Kitapcioglu G, Caymaz-Bor C, Gilbert RJ. Gastroesophageal reflux disease in a low-income region in Turkey. Am J Gastroenterol. 2005;100:759–65.

36. Kitapçioğlu G, Mandiracioğlu A, Caymaz Bor C, Bor S. Overlap of symptoms of dyspepsia and gastroesophageal reflux in the community. Turk J Gastroenterol. 2007;18:14–9.

37. Mungan Z. Prevalence and demographic determinants of gastroesophageal reflux disease (GERD) in the Turkish general population: a population-based cross-sectional study. Turk J Gastroenterol. 2012;23:323–32.

38. Moshkowitz M, Horowitz N, Halpern Z, Santo E. Gastroesophageal reflux disease symptoms: prevalence, sociodemographics and treatment patterns in the adult Israeli population. World J Gastroenterol. 2011;17:1332–5.

39. Sperber AD, Halpern Z, Shvartzman P, , Friger M, Freud T, Neville A, et al. Prevalence of GERD symptoms in a representative Israeli adult population. J Clin Gastroenterol 2007;41:457–461.

40. Pan GXG, Ke M, et al. Epidemiological study of symptomatic gastro-esophageal reflux disease in China: Beijing and Shanghai. Chin J Dig Dis. 2000;1:2–8.

41. Fujimoto K, Iwakiri R, Okamoto K, Oda K, Tanaka A, Tsunada S, et al. Characteristics of gastroesophageal reflux disease in Japan: increased prevalence in elderly women. J Gastroenterol. 2003;38(Suppl 15):3–6.

42. Fujiwara Y, Higuchi K, Shiba M, Watanabe T, Tominaga K, Oshitani N, et al. Association between gastroesophageal flap valve, reflux esophagitis, Barrett's epithelium, and atrophic gastritis assessed by endoscopy in Japanese patients. J Gastroenterol. 2003;38:533–9.

43. Kang MS, Park DI, Oh SY, Yoo TW, Ryu SH, Park JH, et al. Abdominal obesity is an independent risk factor for erosive esophagitis in a Korean population. J Gastroenterol Hepatol. 2007;22:1656–61.

44. Lee HL, Eun CS, Lee OY, Jeon YC, Sohn JH, Han DS, et al. Association between GERD-related erosive esophagitis and obesity. J Clin Gastroenterol. 2008;42:672–5.

45. Tseng PH, Lee YC, Chiu HM, Huang SP, Liao WC, Chen CC, et al. Prevalence and clinical characteristics of Barrett's esophagus in a Chinese general population. J Clin Gastroenterol. 2008;42:1074–9.

46. Kaji M, Fujiwara Y, Shiba M, Kohata Y, Yamagami H, Tanigawa T, et al. Prevalence of overlaps between GERD, FD and IBS and impact on health-related quality of life. J Gastroenterol Hepatol. 2010;25:1151–6.

47. Kim N, Lee SW, Cho SI, Park CG, Yang CH, Kim HS, et al. The prevalence of and risk factors for erosive oesophagitis and non-erosive reflux disease: a nationwide multicentre prospective study in Korea. Aliment Pharmacol Ther. 2008;27:173–85.

48. Noh YW, Jung HK, Kim SE, Jung SA. Overlap of erosive and non-erosive reflux diseases with functional gastrointestinal disorders according to Rome III criteria. J Neurogastroenterol Motil. 2010;16:148–56.

49. Yamagishi H, Koike T, Ohara S, Abe Y, Iijima K, Imatani A, et al. Clinical characteristics of gastroesophageal reflux disease in Japan. Hepato-Gastroenterology. 2009;56:1032–4.

50. Zou D, He J, Ma X, Chen J, Gong Y, Man X, et al. Epidemiology of symptom-defined gastro-esophageal reflux disease and reflux esophagitis: the systematic investigation of gastrointestinal diseases in China (SILC). Scand J Gastroenterol. 2011;46:133–41.

51. Rosaida MS, Goh KL. Gastro-oesophageal reflux disease, reflux oesophagitis and non-erosive reflux disease in a multiracial Asian population: a prospective, endoscopy based study. Eur J Gastroenterol Hepatol. 2004;16:495–501.

52. Rajendra S, Kutty K, Karim N. Ethnic differences in the prevalence of endoscopic esophagitis and Barrett's esophagus: the long and short of it all. Dig Dis Sci. 2004;49:237–42.

53. Ho KY, Chan YH, Kang JY. Increasing trend of reflux esophagitis and decreasing trend of helicobacter pylori infection in patients from a multiethnic Asian country. Am J Gastroenterol. 2005;100:1923–8.

54. Al-Humayed SM, Mohamed-Elbagir AK, Al-Wabel AA, Argobi YA. The changing pattern of upper gastro-intestinal lesions in southern Saudi Arabia: an endoscopic study. Saudi J Gastroenterol. 2010;16:35–7.

55. Koop H, Schepp W, Muller-Lissner S, Madisch A, Micklefield G, Messmann H, et al. Consensus conference of the DGVS on gastroesophageal reflux. Z Gastroenterol. 2005;43:163–4. [Article in German]

56. Shimizu Y, Dobashi K, Kobayashi S, Ohki I, Tokushima M, Kusano M, et al. High prevalence of gastroesophageal reflux disease with minimal mucosal change in asthmatic patients. Tohoku J Exp Med. 2006;209:329–36.

57. Chen MJ, Wu MS, Lin JT, Chang KY, Chiu HM, Liao WC, et al. Gastroesophageal reflux disease and sleep quality in a Chinese population. J Formos Med Assoc. 2009;108:53–60.

58. Fujiwara Y, Kohata Y, Kaji M, Nebiki H, Yamasaki T, Sasaki E, et al. Sleep dysfunction in Japanese patients with gastroesophageal reflux disease: prevalence, risk factors, and efficacy of rabeprazole. Digestion. 2010;81:135–41.

59. Kusano M, Kouzu T, Kawano T, Ohara S. Nationwide epidemiological study on gastro-esophageal reflux disease and sleep disorders in the Japanese population. J Gastroenterol. 2008;43:833–41.

60. Wang GR, Zhang H, Wang ZG, Jiang GS, Guo CH. Relationship between dental ero-sion and respiratory symptoms in patients with gastro-oesophageal reflux disease. J Dent. 2010;38:892–8.

61. Mohd H, Qua CS, Wong CH, Azman W, Goh KL. Non-cardiac chest pain: prevalence of reflux disease and response to acid suppression in an Asian population. J Gastroenterol Hepatol. 2009;24:288–93.

62. Yeh C, Hsu CT, Ho AS, Sampliner RE, Fass R. Erosive esophagitis and Barrett's esophagus in Taiwan: a higher frequency than expected. Dig Dis Sci. 1997;42:702–6.

63. Furukawa N, Iwakiri R, Koyama T, Okamoto K, Yoshida T, Kashiwagi Y, et al. Proportion of reflux esophagitis in 6010 Japanese adults: prospective evaluation by endoscopy. J Gastroenterol. 1999;34:441–4.

64. Inamori M, Togawa J, Nagase H, Abe Y, Umezawa T, Nakajima A, et al. Clinical charac-teristics of Japanese reflux esophagitis patients as determined by Los Angeles classification. J Gastroenterol Hepatol. 2003;18:172–6.

65. Hongo M, Nagasaki Y, Shoji T. Epidemiology of esophageal cancer: orient to occident. Effects of chronology, geography and ethnicity. J Gastroenterol Hepatol. 2009;24:729–35.

66. Tu CH, Lee CT, Perng DS, Chang CC, Hsu CH, Lee YC. Esophageal adenocarcinoma arising from Barrett's epithelium in Taiwan. J Formos Med Assoc. 2007;106:664–8.

67. Kim JH, Rhee PL, Lee JH, Lee H, Choi YS, Son HJ, et al. Prevalence and risk factors of Barrett's esophagus in Korea. J Gastroenterol Hepatol. 2007;22:908–12.

68. Chen MJ, Lee YC, Chiu HM, Wu MS, Wang HP, Lin JT. Time trends of endoscopic and patho-logical diagnoses related to gastroesophageal reflux disease in a Chinese population: eight years single institution experience. Dis Esophagus. 2010;23:201–7.

69. Gadour MO, Ayoola EA. Barrett's oesophagus and oesophageal cancer in Saudi Arabia. Trop Gastroenterol. 1999;20:111–5.

70. Lee IS, Choi SC, Shim KN, Jee SR, Huh KC, Lee JH, et al. Prevalence of Barrett's esopha-gus remains low in the Korean population: nationwide cross-sectional prospective multicenter study. Dig Dis Sci. 2010;55:1932–9.

71. Odemiş B, Ciçek B, Zengin NI, Arhan M, Kacar S, Cengiz C, et al. Barrett's esophagus and endoscopically assessed esophagogastric junction integrity in 1000 consecutive Turkish patients undergoing endoscopy: a prospective study. Dis Esophagus. 2009;22:649–55.

72. Park JJ, Kim JW, Kim HJ, Chung MG, Park SM, Baik GH, et al. The prevalence of and risk factors for Barrett's esophagus in a Korean population: a nationwide multicenter prospective study. J Clin Gastroenterol. 2009;43:907–14.

73. Xiong LS, Cui Y, Wang JP, Wang JH, Xue L, Hu PJ, et al. Prevalence and risk factors of Barrett's esophagus in patients undergoing endoscopy for upper gastrointestinal symptoms. J Dig Dis. 2010;11:83–7.

74. Amarapurkar AD, Vora IM, Dhawan PS. Barrett's esophagus. Indian J Pathol Microbiol. 1998;41:431–5.

75. Wong WM, Lim P, Wong BC. Clinical practice pattern of gastroenterologists, primary care physicians, and otolaryngologists for the management of GERD in the Asia-Pacific region: the FAST survey. J Gastroenterol Hepatol. 2004;19(Suppl 3):S54–60.

76. Miyamoto M, Haruma K, Kuwabara M, Nagano M, Okamoto T, Tanaka M. High incidence of newly-developed gastroesophageal reflux disease in the Japanese community: a 6-year follow-up study. J Gastroenterol Hepatol. 2008;23:393–7.

77. Lee SJ, Song CW, Jeen YT, Chun HJ, Lee HS, Um SH, et al. Prevalence of endoscopic reflux esophagitis among Koreans. J Gastroenterol Hepatol. 2001;16:373–6.

78. Lien HC, Chang CS, Yeh HZ, , Ko CW, Chang HY, Cheng KF, et al. Increasing prevalence of erosive esophagitis among Taiwanese aged 40 years and above: a comparison between two time periods. J Clin Gastroenterol 2009;43:926–932.
79. Song HJ, Choi KD, Jung HY, Lee GH, Jo JY, Byeon JS, et al. Endoscopic reflux esophagitis in patients with upper abdominal pain-predominant dyspepsia. J Gastroenterol Hepatol. 2007;22:2217–21.
80. Sollano JD, Wong SN, Andal-Gamutan T, Chan MM, Carpio RE, Tady CS, et al. Erosive esophagitis in the Philippines: a comparison between two time periods. J Gastroenterol Hepatol. 2007;22:1650–5.
81. Ho KY, Cheung TK, Wong BC. Gastroesophageal reflux disease in Asian countries: disorder of nature or nurture? J Gastroenterol Hepatol. 2006;21:1362–5.
82. Cheung TK, Wong BC, Lam SK. Gastro-oesophageal reflux disease in Asia: birth of a 'new' disease? Drugs. 2008;68:399–406.
83. Netinatsunton N, Attasaranya S, Ovartlarnporn B, , Sangnil S, Boonviriya S, Piratvisuth T. The value of Carlsson-dent questionnaire in diagnosis of gastroesophageal reflux disease in area with low prevalence of gastroesophageal reflux disease. J Neurogastroenterol Motil. 2011;17:164–168.
84. Jung HK. Epidemiology of gastroesophageal reflux disease in Asia: a systematic review. J Neurogastroenterol Motil. 2011;17:14–27.
85. Wai CT, Yeoh KG, Ho KY, Kang JY, Lim SG. Diagnostic yield of upper endoscopy in Asian patients presenting with dyspepsia. Gastrointest Endosc. 2002;56:548–51.
86. Yilmaz N, Tuncer K, Tuncyurek M, Ozütemiz O, Bor S. The prevalence of Barrett's esophagus and erosive esophagitis in a tertiary referral center in Turkey. Turk J Gastroenterol. 2006;17:79–83.
87. Amano Y, Ishimura N, Furuta K, , Takahashi Y, Chinuki D, Mishima Y, et al. Which landmark results in a more consistent diagnosis of Barrett's esophagus, the gastric folds or the palisade vessels? Gastrointest Endosc 2006;64:206–211.
88. Manabe N, Mihara HK, et al. The increasing incidence of reflux esophagitis during the past 20 years in Japan. Gastroenterology. 1999;116:A224.

Reasons for the Rise of Gastroesophageal Reflux Disease in Asia

3

Khean Lee Goh

Abstract

Gastroesophageal reflux disease (GERD) was considered an uncommon disease in Asia in the past but is now a rapidly emerging disease. Various factors underlie this rise, which can be broadly divided into environmental and host genetic factors. Among these factors, the rapid increase in overweight and obesity in the region is probably the most important. Other factors include lifestyle changes which have accompanied "Westernization" of the Asian population, including a change in diet, smoking, alcohol consumption, and physical activity, but these are often hard to measure. A decline in *Helicobacter pylori* infection across the region likely plays an important role as well. Ethnic differences and differences in the rate of rise of GERD between ethnic groups in the region point to a key role for host genetic factors. Genetic polymorphisms which involve the interleukin-1B gene have been reported, but more work needs to be done in this area.

Keywords

Gastroesophageal reflux disease • Rise in disease prevalence • Asia • Ethnic differences • Obesity • *H. pylori* infection • Lifestyle changes

Introduction

Once considered an uncommon disease among Asians [1], gastroesophageal reflux disease (GERD) has increased dramatically over the past two decades in the Asia-Pacific region. Many reasons underlie this change. A better awareness and recognition of the disease by patients and doctors have led to an increase in the diagnosis of

K.L. Goh (✉)
University of Malaya, Kuala Lumpur, Malaysia
e-mail: klgoh56@gmail.com

© Springer India 2018
P. Sharma et al. (eds.), *The Rise of Acid Reflux in Asia*,
DOI 10.1007/978-81-322-0846-4_3

the disease, but most experts feel that there is indeed a "real increase" in the disease in this part of the world [2–4]. The reasons for this increase can be broadly divided into extrinsic, or environmental, and host genetic factors.

Environmental Causes

The increase in GERD in Asia has often been attributed to readily identifiable environmental causes, but scientific evidence to support these has often been lacking (Table 3.1).

Change in Diet

Dietary change has been inevitable with growing affluence in many parts of Asia. An increase in the consumption of dietary fat and protein among Asian populations is well documented [5–8]. The role of diet in the causation of GERD has been widely discussed. El-Serag, in a cross-sectional survey, reported an association between high dietary fat and increased risk of reflux disease [9]. Fox et al. showed a high-fat and high-calorie diet increased the severity and frequency of reflux symptoms [10]. In an earlier study from China, Pan et al. showed that eating "greasy and oily" foods is a cause of reflux symptoms [11]. A recent multicenter Indian Society of Gastroenterology Task Force study showed that consumption of nonvegetarian (with a high animal fat content) and fried foods was an independent predictor of GERD [12]. Physiological studies on healthy volunteers and reflux patients have shown an increased transient lower esophageal sphincter relaxation (TLESR) with ingestion of fatty foods [13–15]. It is important to note that dietary fiber, on the contrary, in the El-Serag et al. study, was shown to be protective against reflux disease.

Table 3.1 Causes of increase in GERD in Asia

	Strength of evidence	
Obesity	+++	For both erosive esophagitis and GERD symptoms with an increase in BMI, increase in abdominal girth and visceral adiposity
High-fat diet	+	Limited studies
Smoking	±	
Alcohol intake	+	Limited studies
Ingestion of carbonated drinks	±	No direct evidence
Ingestion of chilies	±	Conflicting data
Physical inactivity	+	No direct evidence
Disappearing *H. pylori* infection	++	
Host genetic factors	++	Different susceptibility of different Asian races

Key: +++ very strong, ++ strong, + modest, ± inconclusive

What about other types of foods? Spicy foods are the normal fare on many Asian tables. Spicy food incorporating chilies have been universally incriminated as a cause of dyspepsia and acid reflux symptoms. But evidence to refute or support this notion is sparse. Capsaicin, which is the active ingredient of chili, has been shown to induce reflux symptoms [16]. In a review of the influence of diet and reflux symptoms in Korea, a wide range of foods including spicy and fatty foods were found to be associated with reflux symptoms, as were carbonated drinks and coffee [17]. Lim et al. showed that curry provokes acid reflux and reflux symptoms [18]. Gonlachanvit reviewed the literature and wrote that although spicy foods aggravated acute abdominal pain and burning symptoms, spicy food and rice in fact improved GERD symptoms in the longer term [19].

Consumption of carbonated drinks has increased exponentially in many parts of Asia with the rapid urbanization and Westernization of the population, and has been postulated as a cause for the increase in GERD in Asia. Carbonated drinks have been shown to increase the number of TLESRs and to lower the esophageal sphincter pressure [20], but this does not seem to translate to an increase in GERD in the real-life situation [21].

Several other "refluxogenic" foods and drinks that lower the esophageal sphincter pressures have been identified, including chocolate, mint sweets, coffee, and tea. Several Asian studies have shown that consumption of coffee and tea was associated with GERD [12, 17]. However, a recent meta-analysis from Korea did not show a correlation between coffee consumption and GERD [22]. Nonetheless, there has been no marked change in coffee or tea consumption in recent years in the Asian population.

Dietary studies remain difficult to perform in terms of accurate measurement of food intake, and results are therefore often difficult to interpret, with low odds ratio and wide confidence intervals.

Cigarette Smoking and Alcohol Consumption

In several epidemiological studies from Asia, smoking has been shown to be a consistent risk factor for reflux disease among Asians. It is estimated that the risk is at least twofold for smoking [23, 24]. Smoking has been shown to be increasing in the Asia-Pacific region [25]. A decrease in lower sphincter pressures that can occur with long-standing smoking is believed to be the putative mechanism [26, 27].

The association between alcohol consumption and GERD has also been reported in several Asian epidemiological studies. Watanabe et al. showed an association for both cigarette smoking and significant alcohol consumption with GERD [28]. Rosaida and Goh showed a strong association of alcohol intake with both reflux esophagitis and nonerosive reflux disease [29]. Alcohol can similarly lower the esophageal sphincter pressure and has also been shown to sensitize the lower esophageal mucosa in accentuating the pain associated with reflux episodes [30–32]. Alcohol intake has also been shown to be on the rise in the Asia-Pacific region and may be contributing to the observed increase in GERD [33].

Physical Activity

Zheng et al. showed that increased physical activity at work was a risk factor for GERD, while recreational physical activity, conversely, was protective against GERD [24]. However, epidemiological studies have shown a long-term protective effect of exercise [23, 24, 34, 35]. Exercise has actually been shown to increase lower esophageal exposure during exercise. A more sedentary lifestyle associated with a recent change in socioeconomic status and urbanization may have resulted in a decrease in physical activity from a previously predominantly "agricultural-based" lifestyle. This could also indicate that other factors associated with modern living, such as obesity, may be putative, and GERD may not be a direct consequence of a change in physical activity.

An Increase in Body Mass Index and Obesity

Perhaps the most important factor in the emergence of GERD in Asia has been the marked increase in the prevalence of obesity and metabolic syndrome in the region [36]. Obesity has indeed become a major problem in Asians. Recent surveys from China have shown that overweight and obesity affects a significant proportion of the population [37–39]. A recent report from India has also reported a marked increase in BMI in their population [40]. Obesity and its attendant associated diseases such as cardiovascular disease, diabetes mellitus, and nonalcoholic fatty liver have been reported to be on the increase in the Asia-Pacific region [41–43].

In a meta-analysis of published studies, Hampel and colleagues have shown that obesity is associated with increased reflux symptoms, erosive esophagitis, and esophageal adenocarcinoma [44]. Many studies from Asia correlating obesity [45, 46] and metabolic syndrome [46–50] with reflux disease have now been published. In particular, the association between visceral adiposity and central obesity has been consistently significant [47, 51–54].

The mechanisms of disease causation—increased intra-abdominal pressure, impaired gastric emptying, decreased lower esophageal sphincter tone, and an increase in the number of transient lower esophageal sphincter relaxations—have been demonstrated in obese subjects [55–59]. A study by Pandolfino et al. employing sophisticated manometric techniques showed an increase in intragastric pressure as well as gastroesophageal pressure gradients in obese individuals [60].

The "epidemic" of obesity in Asia portends a similar exponential increase in obesity-related disease such as GERD.

Disappearing *H. pylori* Infection

An opposing time trend with a decline in *H .pylori* infection and an increase in GERD has been observed throughout the world, including in the Asia-Pacific region [61, 62]. The putative mechanism is inflammation of the gastric mucosa caused by

H. pylori infection, which results in a decrease in acid secretion and a consequent decline in acid-related diseases including GERD and peptic ulcer disease.

Cross-sectional and case-control studies from Asia have shown a consistent inverse relationship between the prevalence of *H. pylori* and GERD [63–66]. Further support for the role of *H. pylori* infection is shown by a stronger negative association with more virulent strains of *H. pylori* (CagA-positive strains) [67, 68].

Reports on the association between *H. pylori* eradication and GERD have, however, been conflicting. Koike et al. showed an increase in gastric acid with *H. pylori* eradication [69]. Wu et al. showed that *H. pylori* eradication led to more "difficult to treat" cases of GERD [70]. Hamada et al. and Inoue et al. have both shown an increase in incidence of erosive esophagitis after *H. pylori* eradication [71, 72]. However, Kim et al. [73] reported no association with *H. pylori* eradication, and Tsukada et al. found an association only in patients with hiatus hernia [74]. In a meta-analysis of seven randomized controlled trials and five cohort studies, no significant difference in the prevalence of erosive or symptomatic GERD was seen in those patients who had *H. pylori* successfully eradicated and those who had a persistent infection [75].

H. pylori especially with the antral predominant or duodenal ulcer phenotype is associated with an increase in gastric acid secretion. This would normalize with *H. pylori* eradication. On the other hand, the corpus predominant or pangastritis phenotype of *H. pylori* infection is associated with a decrease in gastric acid secretion, and a rebound of acid secretion would occur with *H. pylori* eradication unless irreversible atrophic gastritis has already occurred [76]. This difference in the phenotype of *H. pylori* infection is likely to underlie the variable outcome of *H. pylori* eradication that has been reported.

Host Factors

Ethnic Differences: Genetic Predisposition?

The role of host genetic factors in the pathogenesis of GERD is well shown in two important studies where the prevalence of GERD was higher in monozygotic compared to dizygotic twins [77, 78]. Familial clustering of GERD has also been reported [79]. Several genetic mutations influencing host's inflammatory response, DNA repair, mutagenesis, and esophageal sensory function have been described in association with GERD [80].

In Asia different predisposition to GERD among different ethnicity points to a role of host genetic factors and/or environmental factors such as diet common or peculiar to an ethnic group as putative.

High prevalence for GERD symptoms among Chinese, Japanese, and Koreans indicates that these races may be predisposed to develop GERD in the first place. In a multiracial country like Malaysia, with three major Asian races—Malay, Indian, and Chinese—it is possible to compare changes between these races living in the same environment. Rosaida and Goh identified Indian race as a risk factor for GERD and erosive reflux esophagitis [29]. In another study, Rajendra et al. showed a distinct predisposition to develop Barrett's esophagus in Indian patients and further showed a predominance of HLA B7 subtype among Indians with the disease [81].

Furthermore, genetic predisposition to GERD among different ethnic groups would mean that such an increase would be more prominent among certain racial groups. This has been demonstrated in a time-trend study, where Goh et al. recorded a significantly higher rise in esophagitis over a 10-year interval among Indians (2.4–8.1%) compared to Chinese (1.7–6.4%) and Malays (1.5–3.7%) [62].

In a particular geographical region in Malaysia, environmental influences remain fairly consistent across all races, as much social intermixing (but not intermarriages) in daily life have taken place. The differential increase in the prevalence of GERD between races marks out Indians as a genetically susceptible race to the influence of changing environmental factors in the development of GERD. Interestingly, a study from the UK lends support to this notion by identifying South Asian race (Indian) vs. White Caucasians as a risk factor for GERD [82].

What specific genetic polymorphisms identify predisposition to reflux disease is, however, still not entirely clarified. Reports of interleukin-1B polymorphisms in studies from India, Japan, and Korea have shown a predilection to GERD in subjects with less pro-inflammatory genotypes [83–85]. More substantive work has still to be carried out in this area of research.

Conclusion

The pathogenesis of GERD is a complex interaction between environmental and host factors. The increase in GERD in Asia is the result of several environmental factors, including a marked increase in obesity across the region, and changes in diet and lifestyle of the population interacting with a genetically susceptible population. In a region with a high *H. pylori* prevalence, the declining rates of the infection are likely to also contribute in a significant way to the increased prevalence of GERD in Asia.

References

1. Goh KL, Chang SC, Fock KM, Ke MY, Park HJ, Lam SK. Gastro-esophageal reflux disease in Asia. J Gastroenterol Hepatol. 2000;15:230–8.
2. Cheung TK, Wong BC, Lam SK. Gastro-oesophageal reflux disease in Asia: birth of a 'new' disease? Drugs. 2008;68(4):399–406. Review
3. Ho KY. Gastroesophageal reflux disease in Asia: a condition in evolution. J Gastroenterol Hepatol. 2008 May;23(5):716–22.
4. Goh KL. Gastroesophageal reflux disease in Asia: a historical perspective and present challenges. J Gastroenterol Hepatol. 2011;26(Suppl 1):2–10.
5. Yoshiike N, Matsumura Y, Iwaya M, Sugiyama M, Yamaguchi M. National Nutrition Survey in Japan. J Epidemiol. 1996;6(Suppl 3):S189–200.
6. Kim S, Moon S, Popkin BM. The nutrition transition in South Korea. Am J Clin Nutr. 2000;71:44–53.

7. Ge KY. The dietary and nutritional status of Chinese population 1992. In: National Nutrition Survey. Beijing: People's Medical Publishing House; 1999.
8. Chen C. Fat intake and nutritional status of children in China. Am J Clin Nutr. 2000;72(suppl):1368S–72S.
9. El-Serag HB, Satia JA, Rabeneck L. Dietary intake and the risk of gastro-esophageal reflux disease: a cross sectional study in volunteers. Gut. 2005;54:11–7.
10. Fox M, Barr C, Nolan S, Lomer M, Anggiansah A, Wong T. The effects of dietary fat and calorie density on esophageal acid exposure and reflux symptoms. Clin Gastroenterol Hepatol. 2007;5:439–44.
11. Pan GZ, Xu GM, Ke MY, Han SM, Guo HP, Li ZS, et al. Epidemiological study of symptomatic gastroesophageal reflux disease in China: Beijing and Shanghai. China J Dig Dis. 2000;1:2–8.
12. Bhatia SJ, Reddy DN, Ghoshal UC, Jayanthi V, Abraham P, Choudhuri G, et al. Epidemiology and symptom profile of gastroesophageal reflux in the Indian population: report of the Indian Society of Gastroenterology Task Force. Indian J Gastroenterol. 2011 May;30(3):118–27.
13. Becker DJ, Sinclair J, Castell DO, et al. A comparison of high and low fat meals on postprandial esophageal acid exposure. Am J Gastroenterol. 1989;84:782–6.
14. Nebel OT, Castell DO. Lower esophageal sphincter pressure after food ingestion. Gastroenterology. 1972;63:778–83.
15. Murphy DW, Castell DO. Chocolate and heartburn: evidence of increased esophageal acid exposure after chocolate ingestion. Am J Gastroenterol. 1988;83:633–6.
16. Herrera-López JA, Mejía-Rivas MA, Vargas-Vorackova F, Valdovinos-Díaz MA. Capsaicin induction of esophageal symptoms in different phenotypes of gastroesophageal reflux disease. Rev Gastroenterol Mex. 2010;75:396–404.
17. Song JH, Chung SJ, Lee JH, Kim YH, Chang DK, Son HJ, et al. Relationship between gastroesophageal reflux symptoms and dietary factors in Korea. J Neurogastroenterol Motil. 2011;17:54–60.
18. Lim LG, Tay H, Ho KY. Curry induces acid reflux and symptoms in gastroesophageal reflux disease. Dig Dis Sci. 2011;56:3546–50.
19. Golanchavit S. Are Rice and Spicy Diet Good for Functional Gastrointestinal Disorders? J Neurogastroenterol Motil. 2010;16:131–8.
20. Shukla A, Meshram M, Gopan A, Ganjewar V, Kumar P, Bhatia SJ. Ingestion of a carbonated beverage decreases lower esophageal sphincter pressure and increases frequency of transient lower esophageal sphincter relaxation in normal subjects. Indian J Gastroenterol. 2012;31:121–4.
21. Johnson T, Gerson L, Hershcovici T, Stave C, Fass R. Systematic review: the effects of carbonated beverages on gastro-oesophageal reflux disease. Aliment Pharmacol Ther. 2010;31:607–14.
22. Kim J, Oh SW, Myung SK, Kwon H, Lee C, Yun JM, The Korean Meta-analysis (KORMA) Study Group. Association between coffee intake and gastroesophageal reflux disease: a meta-analysis. Dis Esophagus. 2013;27:311–7.
23. Nilsson M, Johnsen R, Ye W, Hveem K, Lagergren J. Lifestyle related risk factors in the aetiology of gastro-oesophageal reflux. Gut. 2004;53:1730–5.
24. Zheng Z, Nordenstedt H, Pedersen NL, Lagergren J, Ye W. Lifestyle factors and risk for symptomatic gastroesophageal reflux in monozygotic twins. Gastroenterology. 2007;132:87–95.
25. Barzi F, Huxley R, Jamrozik K, Lam TH, Ueshima H, Gu D, et al. Association of smoking and smoking cessation with major causes of mortality in the Asia Pacific Region: the Asia Pacific Cohort Studies Collaboration. Tob Control. 2008;17:166–72.
26. Kahrilas PJ, Gupta RR. Mechanisms of acid reflux associated with cigarette smoking. Gut. 1990;31:4–10.
27. Kadakia SC, Kikendall JW, Maydonovitch C, Johnson LF. Effect of cigarette smoking on gastroesophageal reflux measured by 24-h ambulatory esophageal pH monitoring. Am J Gastroenterol. 1995;90:1785–90.

28. Watanabe Y, Fujiwara Y, Shiba M, Watanabe T, Tominaga K, Oshitani N, et al. Cigarette smoking and alcohol consumption associated with gastro-oesophageal reflux disease in Japanese men. Scand J Gastroenterol. 2003;38:807–11.
29. Rosaida MS. Goh KL Gastro-oesophageal reflux disease, reflux oesophagitis and non-erosive reflux disease in a multiracial Asian population: a prospective, endoscopy based study. Eur J Gastroenterol Hepatol. 2004;16:495–501.
30. Kaufman SE, Kaye MD. Induction of gastro-oesophageal reflux by alcohol. Gut. 1978;19:336–8.
31. Mayer EM, Grabowski CJ, Fisher RS. Effects of graded doses of alcohol upon esophageal motor function. Gastroenterology. 1978;75:1133–6.
32. Bor S, Bor-Caymaz C, Tobey NA, Abdulnour-Nakhoul S, Orlando RC. Esophageal exposure to ethanol increases risk of acid damage in rabbit esophagus. Dig Dis Sci. 1999;44:290–300.
33. Lam TH, Chim D. Controlling Alcohol-Related Global Health Problems. Asia Pac J Public Health. 2010;22:203S–8S.
34. Nocon M, Labenz J, Willich SN. Lifestyle factors and symptoms of gastroesophageal reflux – a population-based study. Aliment Pharmacol Ther. 2006;23:169–74.
35. Nandurkar S, Locke GR 3rd, Fett S, Zinsmeister AR, Cameron AJ, Talley NJ. Relationship between body mass index, diet, exercise and gastro-oesophageal reflux symptoms in a community. Aliment Pharmacol Ther. 2004;20:497–505.
36. Goh KL. Obesity and increasing gastroesophageal reflux disease in Asia. J Gastroenterol Hepatol. 2007;22:1557–8. (editorial)
37. Gu D, Reynolds K, Wu X, Chen J, Duan X, Reynolds RF, et al. Prevalence of the metabolic syndrome and overweight among adults in China. Lancet. 2005;365:1398–405.
38. Wu Y. Overweight and obesity in China. The once lean giant has a weight problem that is increasing rapidly. BMJ. 2006;333:362–3.
39. Wang Y, Mi J, Shan XY, Wang QJ, GE KY. Is China facing an obesity epidemic and the consequences? The trends in obesity and chronic disease in China. Int J Obes. 2007;31:177–88.
40. Wang Y, Chen HJ, Shaikh S, Mathur P. Is obesity becoming a public health problem in India? Examine the shift from under- to overnutrition problems over time. Obes Rev. 2009;10:456–74.
41. Chitturi S, Farrell GC, George J. Non-alcoholic steatohepatitis in the Asia-Pacific region: future shock? J Gastroenterol Hepatol. 2004;19:368–74. Review
42. Li G, Chen X, Jang Y, Wang J, Xing X, Yang W, et al. Obesity, coronary heart disease risk factors and diabetes in Chinese: an approach to the criteria of obesity in the Chinese population. Obes Rev. 2002;3:167–72.
43. Ishikawa-Takata K, Ohta T, Moritaki K, Gotou T, Inoue S. Obesity, weight change and risks for hypertension, diabetes and hypercholesterolemia in Japanese men. Eur J Clin Nutr. 2002;56:601–7.
44. Hampel H, Abraham NS, El-Serag HB. Meta-analysis: obesity and the risk for gastroesophageal reflux disease and its complications. Ann Intern Med. 2005;143:199–211.
45. Kang MS, Park DI, Oh SY, Yoo TW, Ryu SH, Park JH, et al. Abdominal obesity is an independent risk factor for erosive esophagitis in a Korean population. J Gastroenterol Hepatol. 2007;22:1656–61.
46. Nam SY, Choi IJ, Nam BH, Park KW, Kim CG. Obesity and weight gain as risk factors for erosive oesophagitis in men. Aliment Pharmacol Ther. 2009;29:1042–52.
47. Chung SJ, Kim D, Park MJ, Kim YS, Kim JS, Jung HC, et al. Metabolic syndrome and visceral obesity as risk factors for reflux oesophagitis: a cross-sectional case-control study of 7078 Koreans undergoing health check-ups. Gut. 2008;57:1360–5.
48. Moki F, Kusano M, Mizuide M, Shimoyama Y, Kawamura O, Takagi H, et al. Association between reflux oesophagitis and features of the metabolic syndrome in Japan. Aliment Pharmacol Ther. 2007;26:1069–75.
49. Park JH, Park DI, Kim HJ, Cho YK, Sohn CI, Jeon WK, et al. Metabolic syndrome is associated with erosive esophagitis. World J Gastroenterol. 2008;14:5442–7.
50. Chua CS, Lin YM, Yu FC, Hsu YH, Chen JH, Yang KC, et al. Metabolic risk factors associated with erosive esophagitis. J Gastroenterol Hepatol. 2009;24:1375–9.

51. Lee HL, Eun CS, Lee OY, Jeon YC, Han DS, Yoon BC, et al. Association between erosive esophagitis and visceral fat accumulation quantified by abdominal CT scan. J Clin Gastroenterol. 2009;43:240–3.
52. Tai CM, Lee YC, Tu HP, Huang CK, Wu MT, Chang CY, et al. The Relationship Between Visceral Adiposity and the Risk of Erosive Esophagitis in Severely Obese Chinese Patients. Obesity. 2010;18:2165–9.
53. Yasuhara H, Miyake Y, Toyokawa T, Matsumoto K, Takahara M, Imada T, et al. Large waist circumference is a risk factor for reflux esophagitis in Japanese males. Digestion. 2010;81:181–7.
54. Nam SY, Choi IJ, Ryu KH, Park BJ, Kim HB, Nam BH. Abdominal Visceral Adipose Tissue Volume is Associated with Increased Risk of Erosive Esophagitis in Men and Women. Gastroenterology. 2010;139:1902–11.
55. Barak N, Ehrenpreis ED, Harrison JR, Sitrin MD. Gastro-oesophageal reflux disease in obesity: pathophysiological and therapeutic considerations. Obes Rev. 2002;3:9–15.
56. Maddox A, Horowitz M, Wishart J, Collins P. Gastric and oesophageal emptying in obesity. Scand J Gastroenterol. 1989;24:593–8.
57. O'Brien TF Jr. Lower esophageal sphincter pressure (LESP) and esophageal function in obese humans. J Clin Gastroenterol. 1980;2:145–8.
58. Orlando RC. Overview of the mechanisms of gastroesophageal reflux. Am J Med. 2001;111(Suppl 8A):174S–7S.
59. Wu JC, Mui LM, Cheung CM, Chan Y, Sung JJ. Obesity is associated with increased transient lower esophageal sphincter relaxation. Gastroenterology. 2007;132:883–9.
60. Pandolfino JE, El-Serag HB, Zhang Q, Shah N, Ghosh SK, Kahrilas PJ. Obesity: a challenge to esophagogastric junction integrity. Gastroenterology. 2006;130:639–49.
61. Ho KY, Chan YH. el-Kang JY. Increasing trend of reflux esophagitis and decreasing trend of Helicobacter pylori infection in patients from a multiethnic Asian country. Am J Gastroenterol. 2005;100:1923–8.
62. Goh KL, Wong HT, Lim CH, Rosaida MS. Time trends in peptic ulcer, erosive reflux oesophagitis, gastric and oesophageal cancers in a multiracial Asian population. Aliment Pharmacol Ther. 2009;29:774–80.
63. Wu JC, Sung JJ, Ng EK, Go MY, Chan WB, Chan FK, et al. Prevalence and distribution of Helicobacter pylori in gastroesophageal reflux disease: a study from the East. Am J Gastroenterol. 1999;94:1790–4.
64. Haruma K, Hamada H, Mihara M, Kamada T, Yoshihara M, Sumii K, et al. Negative association between Helicobacter pylori infection and reflux esophagitis in older patients: case-control study in Japan. Helicobacter. 2000;5:24–9.
65. Fujishiro H, Adachi K, Kawamura A, Katsube T, Ono M, Yuki M, et al. Influence of Helicobacter pylori infection on the prevalence of reflux esophagitis in Japanese patients. J Gastroenterol Hepatol. 2001;16:1217–21.
66. Rajendra S, Ackroyd R, Robertson IK, Ho JJ, Karim N, Kutty KM. Helicobacter pylori, ethnicity, and the gastroesophageal reflux disease spectrum: a study from the East. Helicobacter. 2007;12:177–83.
67. Vicari JJ, Peek RM, Falk GW, Goldblum JR, Easley KA, Schnell J, et al. The seroprevalence of cagA-positive Helicobacter pylori strains in the spectrum of gastroesophageal reflux disease. Gastroenterology. 1998;115:50–7.
68. Lai CH, Poon SK, Chen YC, Chang CS, Wang WC. Lower prevalence of Helicobacter pylori infection with vacAs1a, cagA-positive, and babA2-positive genotype in erosive reflux esophagitis disease. Helicobacter. 2005;10:577–85.
69. Koike T, Ohara S, Sekine H, Iijima K, Kato K, Toyota T, et al. Increased gastric acid secretion after Helicobacter pylori eradication may be a factor for developing reflux oesophagitis. Aliment Pharmacol Ther. 2001;15:813–20.
70. Wu JC, Chan FK, Ching JY, Leung WK, Hui Y, Leong R, et al. Effect of Helicobacter pylori eradication on treatment of gastro-oesophageal reflux disease: a double blind, placebo controlled, randomised trial. Gut. 2004;53:174–9.

71. Hamada H, Haruma K, Mihara M, Kamada T, Yoshihara M, Sumii K, et al. High incidence of reflux oesophagitis after eradication therapy for Helicobacter pylori: impacts of hiatal hernia and corpus gastritis. Aliment Pharmacol Ther. 2000;14:729–35.

72. Inoue H, Imoto I, Taguchi Y, Kuroda M, Nakamura M, Horiki N, et al. Reflux esophagitis after eradication of Helicobacter pylori is associated with the degree of hiatal hernia. Scand J Gastroenterol. 2004;39:1061–5.

73. Kim N, Lim SH, Lee KH. No protective role of Helicobacter pylori in the pathogenesis of reflux esophagitis in patients with duodenal or benign gastric ulcer in Korea. Dig Dis Sci. 2001;46:2724–32.

74. Tsukada K, Miyazaki T, Katoh H, Fukuchi M, Fukai Y, Kimura H, et al. The incidence of reflux oesophagitis after eradication therapy for Helicobacter pylori. Eur J Gastroenterol Hepatol. 2005;17:1025–8.

75. Yaghoobi M, Farrokhyar F, Yuan Y, Hunt RH. Is there an increased risk of GERD after Helicobacter pylori eradication?: a meta-analysis. Am J Gastroenterol. 2010;105:1007–13.

76. Lee A, Dixon MF, Danon SJ, Kuipers E, Mégraud F, Larsson H, et al. Local acid production and Helicobacter pylori: a unifying hypothesis of gastroduodenal disease. Eur J Gastroenterol Hepatol. 1995;7:461–5. Review

77. Cameron AJ, Lagergren J, Henriksson C, Nyren O, Locke GR 3rd, Pedersen NL. Gastroesophageal reflux disease in monozygotic and dizygotic twins. Gastroenterology. 2002;122:55–9.

78. Mohammed I, Cherkas LF, Riley SA, Spector TD, Trudgill NJ. Genetic influences in gastro-oesophageal reflux disease: a twin study. Gut. 2003;52:1085–9.

79. Trudgill NJ, Kapur KC, Riley SA. Familial clustering of reflux symptoms. Am J Gastroenterol. 1997;94:1172–8.

80. Ghoshal UC, Chourasia D. Genetic factors in the pathogenesis of gastroesophageal reflux disease. Indian J Gastroenterol. 2011 Mar;30(2):55–62.

81. Rajendra S, Kutty K, Karim N. Ethnic differences in the prevalence of endoscopic esophagitis and Barrett's esophagus: the long and short of it all. Dig Dis Sci. 2004;49:237–42.

82. Mohammed I, Nightingale P, Trudgill NJ. Risk factors for gastro-oesophageal reflux disease symptoms: a community study. Aliment Pharmacol Ther. 2005;21:821–7.

83. Muramatsu A, Azuma T, Okuda T, Satomi S, Ohtani M, Lee S, et al. Association between interleukin-1beta-511C/T polymorphism and reflux esophagitis in Japan. J. Gastroenterol. 2005;40:873–7.

84. Chourasia D, Achyut BR, Tripathi S, Mittal B, Mittal RD, Ghoshal UC. Genotypic and functional roles of IL-1B and IL-1RN on the risk of gastroesophageal reflux disease: the presence of IL-1B-511*T/IL-1RN*1 (T1) haplotype may protect against the disease. Am J Gastroenterol. 2009;104:2704–13.

85. Kim JJ, Kim N, Hwang S, Kim JY, Kim JY, Choi YJ, et al. Relationship of interleukin-1β levels and gastroesophageal reflux disease in Korea. J Gastroenterol Hepatol. 2013;28:90–8.

Pathophysiology and Acid Production Different in Asians: Different from the Western People?

Noriaki Manabe and Ken Haruma

Abstract

The prevalence of gastroesophageal reflux disease (GERD) is reported to be more common in Western countries compared to Asian countries. GERD results from an imbalance between aggressive factors such as gastric juice and defensive factors such as esophageal motility, which protect the esophageal mucosa. Of these factors, gastric acid secretion is one of the important aggressive factors and is responsible for the esophageal mucosal damage in GERD. The epidemiological differences in GERD between people in Asia and those in Western countries are partly due to the differences in gastric acid secretion related to gastric mucosal atrophy, *Helicobacter pylori* (*H. pylori*) infection and a westernized lifestyle. In recent times, rapid decline in *H. pylori* infection rates, as well as in severe atrophic gastritis, and an increase in energy intake, especially fatty food, can be observed in many Asian countries. Considering the above trends in Asian countries, we will see a marked increase in the incidence of reflux esophagitis in the future, although it is still unknown whether severe forms of reflux esophagitis including Barrett's esophagitis may also increase, as well as Barrett's esophageal adenocarcinomas. Further research will be necessary to monitor these trends.

Keywords

Gastroesophageal reflux disease • Erosive esophagitis • Epidemiology • Pathophysiology • Asian countries • Western countries • Gastric acid • *Helicobacter pylori* • Atrophic gastritis

N. Manabe (✉)
Division of Endoscopy and Ultrasonography, Department of Clinical Pathology and Laboratory Medicine, Kawasaki Medical School, Kurashiki, Japan
e-mail: n_manabe@hkg.odn.ne.jp

K. Haruma
Department of General Internal Medicine 2, Kawasaki Medical School General Medical Center, Okayama, Japan

© Springer India 2018
P. Sharma et al. (eds.), *The Rise of Acid Reflux in Asia*,
DOI 10.1007/978-81-322-0846-4_4

Introduction

Gastroesophageal reflux disease (GERD) is a condition that develops when reflux of gastric contents causes troublesome symptoms and/or complications [1]. Although GERD is the most common gastrointestinal (GI) disease worldwide, there might be several epidemiological differences in GERD between people in Asian countries and those in Western countries. Differences in these epidemiological data suggest that the pathophysiology of GERD in people in Asian countries might differ from those in Western countries.

Although the pathophysiology of GERD is complex, there is an imbalance between aggressive factors from the stomach contents (gastric acid and duodenal contents) and defensive factors protecting the esophagus (antireflux barriers, esophageal acid clearance, and tissue resistance). Of these several factors, gastric acid secretion is the major offender and is primarily responsible for the esophageal mucosal damage in GERD [2]. These differences are partly due to the differences in gastric acid secretion. For example, the gastric acid secretion of the Japanese is reportedly lower than that of Western people. Furthermore, *Helicobacter pylori* (*H. pylori*) is also an important pathogen known to be associated with atrophic gastritis, peptic ulcer, gastric carcinoma, and mucosa-associated lymphoid tissue lymphoma [3]. Gastric acid secretion is known to decrease with the progression of atrophic gastritis [4]. Therefore, we cannot ignore the influence of *H. pylori* infection when we discuss the role of gastric acid secretion in the pathophysiology of GERD.

In this chapter, we will review the differences in and pathophysiology of GERD between people in Asian countries and those in Western countries, mainly from the viewpoint of gastric acid secretion.

Differences in Clinical Characteristics of GERD Between East and West

Epidemiology: Prevalence of GERD

GERD is prevalent in Western countries such as the United Kingdom and United States, where the prevalence of monthly heartburn has been reported to be about 29–44% [5]. Reflux esophagitis also accounts for a significant proportion of upper GI endoscopic findings in these countries. On the other hand, GERD is considered to be less prevalent, and endoscopic severity of reflux esophagitis appears to be milder in Asian countries [2].

The prevalence of GERD differs depending on whether the analysis is based on symptoms (primarily heartburn) or endoscopic findings (esophagitis of the disease).

Symptom-Based Prevalence of GERD
In a nationwide population-based study by the Gallup Organization in 1998 in the United States [6], 44% of people reported heartburn at least once a month. More

convincing data obtained by Locke and colleagues [7] revealed that the prevalence of heartburn and regurgitation in the previous 12 months were noted to be 42 and 45%, respectively; frequent symptoms (at least once a week) were reported by 20% of respondents. Variable prevalence rates for symptomatic GERD have been reported from Europe, ranging from 5% in Switzerland to 27% in Finland [8].

On the other hand, most Asian community-based studies for the symptom-based prevalence of GERD (at least weekly heartburn or regurgitation) have been reported to be generally less than 10% [9, 10].

The difference in the prevalence of symptom-based GERD between people in Asian countries and those in Western countries comes from a variety of factors. The first factor is the lower prevalence of patients with GERD in Asian countries. The second factor is the difference in the recognition of the meaning of "heartburn." Spechler et al. [11] reported that Asian GERD patients seldom complained of heartburn, and many of them poorly understood the meaning of the term. This probably contributed to the underdiagnosis of GERD. The third factor for the under-recognition of GERD among Asian doctors is the tendency for GERD to present atypically. Noncardiac chest pain [12], globus sensation [13], and asthma [14] are not uncommon manifestations of GERD in Asian patients, often without associated heartburn and/or acid regurgitation [12].

Endoscopy-Based Prevalence of GERD

Erosive esophagitis is a common finding among Western patients with GERD. A single endoscopist compared consecutive patients with upper abdominal discomfort seen personally in England with an equal number of patients seen in Singapore and found reflux esophagitis in 25% of English patients but in only 6% of Singaporean patients [15]. In tandem with lesser frequency, the severity of erosive esophagitis in Asian patients is also mild. Several endoscopic studies in Taiwan and Korea showed that the prevalence of endoscopic esophagitis ranged from 3.4 to 9% among participants in health checkup programs, and more than 80% of these had mild esophagitis [16]. Recent Japanese endoscopic studies report an overall proportion of erosive esophagitis at 14 to 16%, [17] which is equivalent to that reported in Western countries (Fig. 4.1) [16].

Causes of GERD

The pathophysiology of GERD is complex and results from an imbalance between aggressive factors from gastric contents (gastric acidity, volume, and duodenal contents) and defensive factors protecting the esophageal mucosa (antireflux barriers, esophageal acid clearance, and tissue resistance) (Fig. 4.2). The pathophysiological mechanisms of GERD in Asian patients are similar to those in Western populations [18].

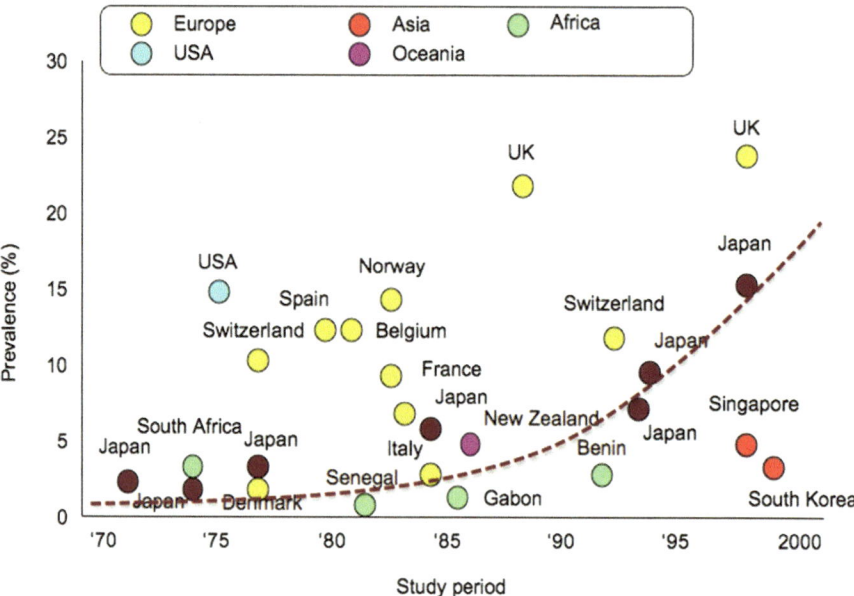

Fig. 4.1 Prevalence of GERD in the world in relation to the study period. Colors represent regions in the world, with *yellow* indicating Europe, *red* Asia, *green* Africa, *blue* the United States, and *pink* Oceania. The prevalence of GERD in relation to the study period in Japan is shown in the color of *Indian red*. The prevalence of GERD in Japan began to increase from the end of the 1990s

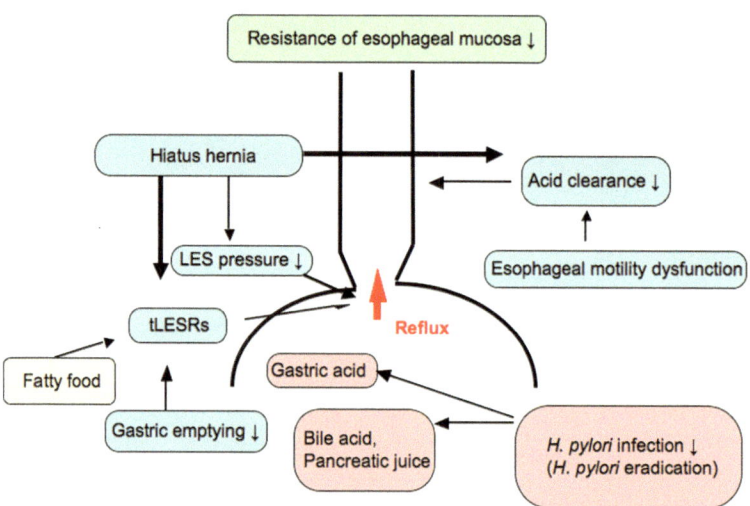

Fig. 4.2 The pathophysiology of GERD. tLESRs, transient lower esophageal sphincter relaxations; *LES*, lower esophageal sphincter; *H. pylori, Helicobacter pylori*. GERD results from an imbalance between aggressive factors from gastric contents (gastric acidity, volume, and duodenal contents) and defensive factors protecting the esophageal mucosa (antireflux barriers, esophageal acid clearance, and tissue resistance)

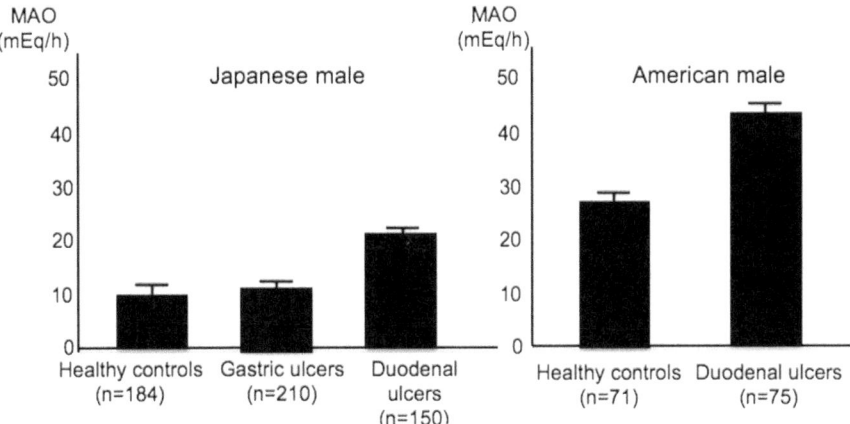

Fig. 4.3 Maximal acid output between Japanese male and American male. *MAO*, maximal acid output

Aggressive Factors

The aggressive factors are more important than defensive factors; decrease in gastric acid secretion induced by atrophic gastritis prevents acid reflux, even though defensive factors such as the esophageal motor dysfunction are impaired. Previous studies show that the total percentage of time that the pH is below 4.0 is higher in GERD patients than in healthy controls, and its value increases according to the endoscopic severity of erosive esophagitis [19].

Gastric contents contain a variety of noxious agents, including acid and pepsin. When defensive factors are unable to cope with these contents, esophageal cell damage and pain can occur. Hydrochloric acid present in the gastric contents exerts cell-damaging effects by disturbing the pH/ ion balance [20]. Proteolytic enzymes such as pepsin and trypsin can disrupt epithelial structures by digesting cell surfaces and promoting cell shredding [21]. Indeed, pepsin is thought to be the major cause of heartburn and erosive esophagitis, but only in combination with acid, as it is inactive when the pH is greater than 4. On the other hand, acid alone may cause little damage except at very high concentrations (pH < 2) [22].

The gastric acid secretion among Japanese [23], Chinese [24], and Indian [25] subjects is reportedly lower than that of Western people. Haruma et al. found that maximal acid output of Japanese men was almost half as compared to that of American men, regardless of whether they suffered from duodenal ulcer disease or not (Fig. 4.3) [23]. In an earlier study, Lam et al. [24] found that the maximal acid output was higher in Scots than in the Chinese for both controls and duodenal ulcer patients. Although the reasons for these differences in the gastric acid output between people in Asian countries and Western countries are not known in detail, there might be several explanations like differences in the rate of *H. pylori* infection, dietary habits, and body mass index between people in the East and those in the West.

Gastric acid secretion is known to be lower in patients with *H. pylori* infection. *H. pylori* infection causes atrophic gastritis that causes a decrease in acid secretion. Therefore, acid secretion might not be sufficient to cause erosive esophagitis, even if their esophageal motor functions, including antireflux barrier and esophageal motility, are impaired [26–28]. That is one explanation for why the prevalence of moderate to severe forms of erosive esophagitis among Asian patients is not as high as in people in Western countries.

Defensive Factors

The defensive factors for protecting the esophageal mucosa from refluxate from the stomach are the antireflux barriers. This is an anatomically complex region that includes the intrinsic lower esophageal sphincter (LES), the diaphragmatic crura, the intra-abdominal location of the LES, the phrenoesophageal ligaments, and the acute angle of His (acute angle created between the cardia at the entrance to the stomach and the esophagus). In the past, LES pressure was considered to be important: decreased LES resting pressure and a shorter LES length are associated with increased reflux. These can be caused by physiological factors such as respiration, gastric activity, and body position, as well as hormones, medication, and certain foods. However, recent studies showed that not only resting LES pressure but also patterns of reflux such as transient LES relaxations (tLESRs), free reflux, or strain reflux are important for the pathophysiology of GERD [30].

For the majority of people, reflux episodes occurring during spontaneous relaxations known as tLESRs are not induced by swallowing or peristalsis [30, 31]. The few reflux episodes experienced by healthy individuals are almost always associated with tLESRs [31]. Although individuals with GERD do not have more frequent tLESRs than healthy individuals, [32, 33] tLESRs in individuals with GERD appear to be more likely associated with acid reflux [34, 35]. Hayashi et al. [36] showed that mechanisms of gastroesophageal reflux were similar to those reported in Western countries. However, the rate of acid reflux during tLESRs in GERD patients is higher than in healthy subjects; also, the rates of acid reflux are low as compared to rates reported in Western countries.

Other defensive factors, such as acid clearance including esophageal body function and/or salivary secretion, are also important in the pathophysiology of GERD. Once refluxate has entered the esophagus, the main defense against esophageal damage is secondary peristalsis (mechanical clearance) in the esophagus, which is stimulated by reflux episodes and food boluses and removes around 90% of the refluxate volume [30, 37]. Chemical clearance in the form of salivary bicarbonate neutralizes the acidic pH. Increased esophageal acid exposure in patients with reflux esophagitis could be attributed to impaired esophageal clearance mechanisms. Esophageal transit has been shown to be delayed in patients with GERD [38]. There does not appear to be a difference between individuals with and without esophagitis. It is, however, unclear whether slowed peristalsis is a cause or consequence of repeated acid injury. Manabe et al. showed that esophageal motility dysfunction that caused the abnormality of acid clearance was observed in approximately half of patients with reflux esophagitis and appeared unrelated to the severity of

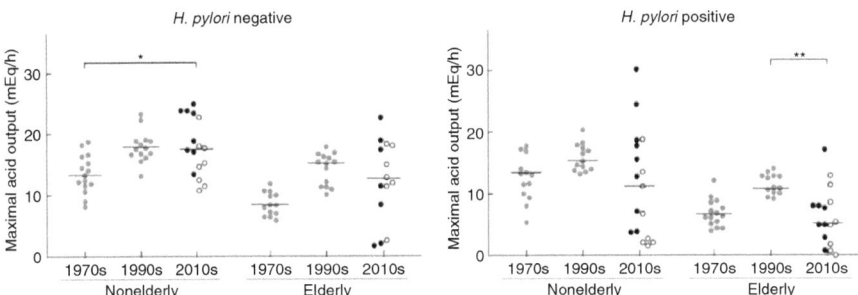

Fig. 4.4 Maximal acid output in the four groups. Each *dot* represents a single case. *Horizontal lines* indicate medians of individual groups (Reprinted from Norihisa Ishimura, No increase in gastric acid secretion in healthy Japanese over the past two decades. Journal of Gastroenterology, Jan 1, 2014;50(8). With permission from Springer)

endoscopically demonstrated erosions [39]. Similar findings were reported from Taiwan [40]. A study from Hong Kong has also shown that in comparable groups of patients with reflux esophagitis, *H. pylori*-infected patients have more severe esophageal dysmotility as compared to noninfected patients. This may contribute to the development of GERD symptoms [41].

Recently research focused on the esophageal mucosal integrity has been intensely undertaken. Esophageal mucosal dilated intercellular spaces (DIS) are frequently observed in patients with GERD and patients with esophagitis [42]. DIS occurs in parallel with a drop in potential difference, diminished transepithelial resistance, and increased esophageal mucosal permeability. It can be caused by acid reflux, but bile acids in the refluxate and/or psychological stress can modulate the development or persistence of DIS [43].

Gastric Acid and GERD

Ishimura et al. [44] found that the acid-secreting capacity, as measured by basal and stimulated gastric acid secretion, of Japanese people has increased over 20 years (1970–1990). This increase in acid secretion was found not only in individuals with *H. pylori* infection but also in those without (Fig. 4.4). Subjects with *H. pylori* infection tended to have lower gastric acid secretion in comparison with those without infection, particularly in elderly subjects.

The mechanism of increased acid secretion in Asians may be due to two different mechanisms. One mechanism is a decreased rate of *H. pylori* infection in Asia [45]. The other mechanism is an increase in gastric acid secretion that may be related to the recent changes in dietary habits and obesity among Asians. For example, fish oil, which was reported to inhibit gastric acid secretion, is now consumed less frequently in Japan [46]. Obesity is on the rise in Asia. In a recent consensus on the relationship between obesity and gastrointestinal diseases, Koh et al. observed that obesity is increasing in most Asian countries [47]. Overweight and obesity increased from 16.7% in 1976–1980 to 24.0% in 2000 in Japan and from 3.7% in 1982 to 19.0% in 2002 in China [48]. This increase in obesity is associated with an increase in the prevalence of erosive esophagitis in Asia, as shown in studies from Korea [49], Japan [50], and China [51].

Helicobacter pylori and GERD

Helicobacter pylori infection decreases gastric acid secretion by causing atrophic gastritis [52]. Although the prevalence of *H. pylori* is steadily decreasing in industrialized nations, probably due to improved hygiene and socioeconomic factors, approximately 50% of the world's population is still colonized with *H. pylori*. In Asia, there is a geographic variation in the seroprevalence rates of *H. pylori* infection. In general, the seroprevalence rates in less developed or developing countries are more than 50%. Among East Asian countries, the overall seroprevalence rate ranges from 58% in China to 39% in Japan. Among Southeast Asian countries, the reported seroprevalence rate is 36% in Malaysia, 31% in Singapore, and 57% in Thailand [54].

Recent epidemiological studies have shown that *H. pylori* infection, especially that with cytotoxin-associated gene A (*cag*A)-positive strain, has a protective effect against the development of GERD and its complications, such as Barrett's esophagitis or esophageal adenocarcinoma [54]. In Japan, Koike et al. [55] showed that *H. pylori* infection was present in 34.3% patients with erosive esophagitis and in 76.2% control subjects (OR 0.163, 95% CI 0.09–0.29). Overall acid secretion was higher in patients with esophagitis. Among *H. pylori*-positive patients, acid secretion was higher in patients with esophagitis as compared to those without esophagitis. Chourasia et al. [56] from India showed that patients with *H. pylori* infection had lower level of gastric acid and less severe reflux. Low gastrin-17, higher age, hiatus hernia, and the absence of *H. pylori* were the best predictors for erosive esophagitis.

Earlier studies showed that *H. pylori* infection in Japan was very low in children under 10 years old (~5%) but was higher among individuals born before 1950 [57]. Subsequently, Fujisawa et al. [45] reported that the prevalence of *H. pylori* antibodies in a group of Japanese people was 72.7% (CI 95%, 68.0–77.3) in 1974, 54.6% (CI 95%, 49.1–60.0) in 1984, and 39.3% (CI 95%, 34.1–44.4) in 1994. Changes in the environmental hygiene after World War II may be related to the decreasing prevalence of *H. pylori* infection in Japan.

The prevalence of *H. pylori* infection in patients with reflux esophagitis negatively correlates with the severity of the disease, i.e., the prevalence of *H. pylori* infection in patients with mild and severe reflux esophagitis was lower than that in healthy controls [58]. Only 10.5% of a cohort of Japanese patients with reflux esophagitis progressed to more severe grade of esophagitis, and none developed Barrett's esophagus over a follow-up of 2–9 years [59].

Also, *H. pylori* infection is less common, and atrophic gastritis is less severe, in patients with reflux esophagitis than in those without the disease [60]. Therefore, it has been hypothesized that *H. pylori*-associated atrophic gastritis protects against reflux esophagitis. Studies in Japan [27, 61] have shown that advanced age, male gender, smoking, absence of severe gastric mucosal atrophy, presence of esophageal hiatal hernia, and high body mass index were associated with reflux esophagitis. Considering that *H. pylori* infection is declining in *Asia*, a marked increase in the prevalence and severity of reflux esophagitis including Barrett's esophagus may occur.

In Western countries, results of studies evaluating the prevalence of *H. pylori* infection in patients with GERD are inconsistent, with some reporting an increased prevalence [62] and others suggesting a decreased prevalence [63]. When the severity of reflux esophagitis is considered, data consistently suggest that patients with more severe esophagitis, including Barrett's esophagitis, have a lower prevalence of *H. pylori* infection rate than healthy controls. Data from seven studies conducted in Europe, the United States, and Japan showed that the overall prevalence of *H. pylori* infection rate in patients with Barrett's esophagitis was 23.5% (range 29–41%) compared with 34.5% (range 29–41%) in patients with less severe forms of reflux esophagitis and 52.3% (range 28.4–76%) in healthy controls [64–68]. Another explanation for the discrepancy between Asian countries and Western countries may be based on the presence of severe gastric mucosal atrophy, not simply by the status of *H. pylori* infection.

Summary

When based on symptoms, GERD is reported to be more common in Western countries compared to Asian countries. Furthermore, among erosive esophagitis, moderate to severe forms of erosive esophagitis is reported to be more common in Western countries. These epidemiological differences between the two areas suggest that the pathophysiology of GERD in Asian countries differs from that in Western countries. So far, three possible reasons or mechanisms are inferred as follows: increase in gastric acid secretion partly due to changes in dietary habits to Western style, the decrease in *H. pylori* infection, and more attention being paid to GERD as well as advanced high-resolution endoscopic imaging. Considering the above trends in Asian countries, we will see a rapid decline in *H. pylori* infection rates in Asian countries in the future, associated with a marked increase in the incidence of reflux esophagitis, although it is still unknown whether severe forms of reflux esophagitis including Barrett's esophagitis and Barrett's esophageal adenocarcinomas may also increase.

References

1. Vakil N, van Zanten SV, Kahrilas P, Dent J, Jones R. Global consensus group. The Montreal definition and classification of gastroesophageal reflux disease: a global evidence-based consensus. Am J Gastroenterol. 2006;101:1900–20.

2. Thomson AB, Chiba N, Armstrong D, Tougas G, Hunt RH. The second Canadian Gastroesophageal reflux disease consensus: moving forward to new concepts. Can J Gastroenterol. 1998;12:551–6.
3. Kawaguchi H, Haruma K, Komoto K, Yoshihara M, Sumii K, Kajiyama G. Helicobacter pylori infection is the major risk factor for atrophic gastritis. Am J Gastroenterol. 1996;91:959–62.
4. Kekki M, Samloff IM, Ihamäki T, Varis K, Siurala M. Age- and sex-related behaviour of gastric acid secretion at the population level. Scand J Gastroenterol. 1982;17:737–43.
5. Drossman DA, Li Z, Andruzzi E, Temple RD, Talley NJ, Thompson WG, et al. U.S. householder survey of functional gastrointestinal disorders. Prevalence, sociodemography, and health impact. Dig Dis Sci. 1993;38:1569–80.
6. Gallup Organisation. A Gallup survey on heartburn across America. Princeton: The Gallop Organization; 1998.
7. Locke GR 3rd, Talley NJ, Fett SL, Zinsmeister AR, Melton LJ 3rd. Prevalence and clinical spectrum of gastroesophageal reflux: a population-based study in Olmsted County, Minnesota. Gastroenterology. 1997;112:1448–56.
8. Stanghellini V. Three-month prevalence rates of gastrointestinal symptoms and the influence of demographic factors: results from the domestic/international gastroenterology surveillance study (DIGEST). Scand J Gastroenterol Suppl. 1999;231:20–8.
9. Dent J, El-Serag HB, Wallander MA, Johansson S. Epidemiology of gastro-oesophageal reflux disease: a systematic review. Gut. 2005;54:710–7.
10. Kang JY. Systematic review: geographical and ethnic differences in gastro-oesophageal reflux disease. Aliment Pharmacol Ther. 2004;20:705–17.
11. Spechler SJ, Jain SK, Tendler DA, Parker RA. Racial differences in the frequency of symptoms and complications of gastro-oesophageal reflux disease. Aliment Pharmacol Ther. 2002;16:1795–800.
12. Yu HK, Tseng CC, Chang CS, Chen GH. Ambulatory 24-hour esophageal manometry and pH-metry in patients with noncardiac chest pain, but no reflux symptoms. Kaohsiung J Med Sci. 1997;13:293–300.
13. Tsutsui H, Manabe N, Uno M, Imamura H, Kamada T, Kusunoki H, et al. Esophageal motor dysfunction plays a key role in GERD with globus sensation–analysis of factors promoting resistance to PPI therapy. Scand J Gastroenterol. 2012;47:893–9.
14. Nakase H, Itani T, Mimura J, Kawasaki T, Komori H, Tomioka H, et al. Relationship between asthma and gastro-oesophageal reflux: significance of endoscopic grade of reflux oesophagitis in adult asthmatics. J Gastroenterol Hepatol. 1999;14:715–22.
15. Kang JY, Ho KY. Different prevalences of reflux oesophagitis and hiatus hernia among dyspeptic patients in England and Singapore. Eur J Gastroenterol Hepatol. 1999;11:845–50.
16. Rasmussen CW. A new endoscopic classification of chronic esophagitis. Am J Gastroenterol. 1976;65:409–15.
17. Inamori M, Togawa J, Nagase H, Abe Y, Umezawa T, Nakajima A, et al. Clinical characteristics of Japanese reflux esophagitis patients as determined by Los Angeles classification. J Gastroenterol Hepatol. 2003;18:172–6.
18. Wu JC. Gastroesophageal reflux disease: an Asian perspective. J Gastroenterol Hepatol. 2008;23:1785–93.
19. Hietanen E, Raitakari OT, Backman H. Validity of ambulatory 24-h oesophageal pH measurement in the diagnosis of reflux disease. Clin Physiol. 1995;15:491–8.
20. Orlando RC, Bryson JC, Powell DW. Mechanisms of H+ injury in rabbit esophageal epithelium. Am J Phys. 1984;246(6 Pt 1):G718–24.
21. Salo JA, Lehto VP, Kivilaakso E. Morphological alterations in experimental esophagitis. Light microscopic and scanning and transmission electron microscopic study. Dig Dis Sci. 1983;28:440–8.
22. Vaezi MF, Singh S, Richter JE. Role of acid and duodenogastric reflux in esophageal mucosal injury: a review of animal and human studies. Gastroenterology. 1995;108:1897–907.
23. Haruma K, Honda K, Kamada T. Reflux esophagitis-Japan and western countries. (in Japanese). Nippon Rinsho. 2004;62:1415–9.

24. Lam SK, Hasan M, Sircus W, Wong J, Ong GB, Prescott RJ. Comparison of maximal acid output and gastrin response to meals in Chinese and Scottish normal and duodenal ulcer subjects. Gut. 1980;21:324–8.
25. Desai HG. Factors affecting maximal acid secretion. Postgrad Med J. 1969;45:272–8.
26. Grande L, Lacima G, Ros E, Pera M, Ascaso C, Visa J, et al. Deterioration of esophageal motility with age: a manometric study of 79 healthy subjects. Am J Gastroenterol. 1999;94:1795–801.
27. Deprez P, Fiasse R. Healing of severe esophagitis improves esophageal peristaltic dysfunction. Dig Dis Sci. 1999;44:125–33.
28. Amano K, Adachi K, Katsube T, Watanabe M, Kinoshita Y. Role of hiatus hernia and gastric mucosal atrophy in the development of reflux esophagitis in the elderly. J Gastroenterol Hepatol. 2001;16:132–6.
29. Herregods TV, Bredenoord AJ, Smout AJ. Pathophysiology of gastroesophageal reflux disease: new understanding in a new era. Neurogastroenterol Motil. 2015;27:1202–13.
30. Dent J, Dodds WJ, Friedman RH, Sekiguchi T, Hogan WJ, Arndorfer RC, et al. Mechanism of gastroesophageal reflux in recumbent asymptomatic human subjects. J Clin Invest. 1980;65:256–67.
31. Dodds WJ, Dent J, Hogan WJ, Helm JF, Hauser R, Patel GK, et al. Mechanisms of gastroesophageal reflux in patients with reflux esophagitis. N Engl J Med. 1982;307:1547–52.
32. Trudgill NJ, Riley SA. Transient lower esophageal sphincter relaxations are no more frequent in patients with gastroesophageal reflux disease than in asymptomatic volunteers. Am J Gastroenterol. 2001;96:2569–74.
33. Wong WM, Lai KC, Hui WM, Hu WH, Huang JQ, Wong NY, et al. Pathophysiology of gastroesophageal reflux diseases in Chinese–role of transient lower esophageal sphincter relaxation and esophageal motor dysfunction. Am J Gastroenterol. 2004;99:2088–93.
34. Mittal RK, McCallum RW. Characteristics and frequency of transient relaxations of the lower esophageal sphincter in patients with reflux esophagitis. Gastroenterology. 1988;95:593–9.
35. Mittal RK, Holloway RH, Penagini R, Blackshaw LA, Dent J. Transient lower esophageal sphincter relaxation. Gastroenterology. 1995;109:601–10.
36. Hayashi Y, Iwakiri K, Kotoyori M, Sakamoto C. Mechanisms of acid gastroesophageal reflux in the Japanese population. Dig Dis Sci. 2008;53:1–6.
37. Orlando RC. Pathophysiology of gastroesophageal reflux disease: esophageal epithelial resistance. In: Castell DO, Richter JE, editors. The esophagus. 4th ed. Philadelphia: Lippincott Williams & Wilkins; 2004. p. 421–33.
38. Eriksen CA, Cullen PT, Sutton D, Kennedy N, Cuschieri A. Abnormal esophageal transit in patients with typical reflux symptoms but normal endoscopic and pH profiles. Am J Surg. 1991;161:657–61.
39. Manabe N, Haruma K, Hata J, Nakamura K, Tanaka S, Chayama K. Autonomic nerve dysfunction is closely associated with the abnormalities of esophageal motility in reflux esophagitis. Scand J Gastroenterol. 2003;38:159–63.
40. Lei WY, Liu TT, Yi CH, Chen CL. Disease characteristics in non-erosive reflux disease with and without endoscopically minimal change esophagitis: are they different? Digestion. 2012;85:27–32.
41. Wu JC, Lai AC, Wong SK, Chan FK, Leung WK, Sung JJ. Dysfunction of oesophageal motility in helicobacter pylori-infected patients with reflux oesophagitis. Aliment Pharmacol Ther. 2001;15:1913–9.
42. Orlando LA, Orlando RC. Dilated intercellular spaces as a marker of GERD. Curr Gastroenterol Rep. 2009;11:190–4.
43. van Malenstein H, Farré R, Sifrim D. Esophageal dilated intercellular spaces (DIS) and nonerosive reflux disease. Am J Gastroenterol. 2008;103:1021–8.
44. Ishimura N, Owada Y, Aimi M, Oshima T, Kamada T, Inoue K, Mikami H, Takeuchi T, Miwa H, Higuchi K, Kinoshita Y. No increase in gastric acid secretion in healthy Japanese over the past two decades. J Gastroenterol. 2015;50:844–52.

45. Fujisawa T, Kumagai T, Akamatsu T, Kiyosawa K, Matsunaga Y. Changes in seroepidemiological pattern of helicobacter pylori and hepatitis a virus over the last 20 years in Japan. Am J Gastroenterol. 1999;94:2094–9.
46. Riber C, Wøjdemann M, Bisgaard T, Ingels H, Rehfeld JF, Olsen O. Fish oil reduces gastric acid secretion. Scand J Gastroenterol. 1999;34:845–8.
47. Koh JC, Loo WM, Goh KL, Sugano K, Chan WK, Chiu WY, et al. Asian consensus on the relationship between obesity and gastrointestinal and liver diseases. J Gastroenterol Hepatol. 2016;31:1405–13.
48. World Health Organization. WHO global database on body mass index. 2015 [cited 1 Apr 2015]. Available from: http://apps.who.int/bmi/index.jsp
49. Nam S, Choi I, Ryu K, Park B, Kim H, Nam B-H. Abdominal visceral adipose tissue volume is associated with increased risk of erosive esophagitis in men and women. Gastroenterology. 2010;139:1902–11.
50. Gunji T, Sato H, Iijima K, et al. Risk factors for erosive esophagitis: a cross-sectional study of a large number of Japanese males. J Gastroenterol. 2011;46:448–55.
51. Tai C, Lee Y, Tu H, et al. The relationship between visceral adiposity and the risk of erosive esophagitis in severely obese Chinese patients. Obesity. 2010;18:2165–9.
52. Katelaris PH, Seow F, Lin BP, Napoli J, Ngu MC, Jones DB. Effect of age, helicobacter pylori infection, and gastritis with atrophy on serum gastrin and gastric acid secretion in healthy men. Gut. 1993;34:1032–7.
53. Fock KM, Ang TL. Epidemiology of helicobacter pylori infection and gastric cancer in Asia. J Gastroenterol Hepatol. 2010;25:479–86.
54. Weston AP, Badr AS, Topalovski M, Cherian R, Dixon A, Hassanein RS. Prospective evaluation of the prevalence of gastric helicobacter pylori infection in patients with GERD, Barrett's esophagus, Barrett's dysplasia, and Barrett's adenocarcinoma. Am J Gastroenterol. 2000;95:387–94.
55. Koike T, Ohara S, Sekine H, Iijima K, Abe Y, Kato K, et al. Helicobacter pylori infection prevents erosive reflux oesophagitis by decreasing gastric acid secretion. Gut. 2001;49:330–4.
56. Chourasia D, Misra A, Tripathi S, Krishnani N, Ghoshal UC. Patients with helicobacter pylori infection have less severe gastroesophageal reflux disease: a study using endoscopy, 24-hour gastric and esophageal pH metry. Indian J Gastroenterol. 2011;30:12–21.
57. Asaka M, Kimura T, Kudo M, Takeda H, Mitani S, Miyazaki T, et al. Relationship of helicobacter pylori to serum pepsinogens in an asymptomatic Japanese population. Gastroenterology. 1992;102:760–6.
58. Shirota T, Kusano M, Kawamura O, Horikoshi T, Mori M, Sekiguchi T. Helicobacter pylori infection correlates with severity of reflux esophagitis: with manometry findings. J Gastroenterol. 1999;34:553–9.
59. Manabe N, Yoshihara M, Sasaki A, Tanaka S, Haruma K, Chayama K. Clinical characteristics and natural history of patients with low-grade reflux esophagitis. J Gastroenterol Hepatol. 2002;17:949–54.
60. Koike T, Ohara S, Sekine H, Iijima K, Kato K, Shimosegawa T, et al. Helicobacter pylori infection inhibits reflux esophagitis by inducing atrophic gastritis. Am J Gastroenterol. 1999;94:3468–72.
61. Fujiwara Y, Higuchi K, Shiba M, Yamamori K, Watanabe Y, Sasaki E, et al. Differences in clinical characteristics between patients with endoscopy-negative reflux disease and erosive esophagitis in Japan. Am J Gastroenterol. 2005;100:754–8.
62. Schenk BE, Kuipers EJ, Klinkenberg-Knol EC, Eskes SA, Meuwissen SG. Helicobacter pylori and the efficacy of omeprazole therapy for gastroesophageal reflux disease. Am J Gastroenterol. 1999;94:884–7.
63. Raghunath A, Hungin AP, Wooff D, Childs S. Prevalence of helicobacter pylori in patients with gastro-oesophageal reflux disease: systematic review. BMJ. 2003;326:737.
64. Haruma K, Hamada H, Mihara M, Kamada T, Yoshihara M, Sumii K, et al. Negative association between helicobacter pylori infection and reflux esophagitis in older patients: case-control study in Japan. Helicobacter. 2000;5:24–9.

65. Vicari JJ, Peek RM, Falk GW, Goldblum JR, Easley KA, Schnell J, et al. The seroprevalence of cagA-positive helicobacter pylori strains in the spectrum of gastroesophageal reflux disease. Gastroenterology. 1998;115:50–7.
66. Kiltz U, Baier J, Schmidt WE, Adamek RJ, Pfaffenbach B. Barrett's metaplasia and helicobacter pylori infection. Am J Gastroenterol. 1999;94:1985–6.
67. Vaezi MF, Falk GW, Peek RM, Vicari JJ, Goldblum JR, Perez-Perez GI, et al. CagA-positive strains of helicobacter pylori may protect against Barrett's esophagus. Am J Gastroenterol. 2000;95:2206–11.
68. Loffeld RJ, Ten Tije BJ, Arends JW. Prevalence and significance of helicobacter pylori in patients with Barrett's esophagus. Am J Gastroenterol. 1992;87:1598–600.

Diagnosis of GERD: Clinical, pH, and Impedance—What Is the Best Approach?

Hiroto Miwa, Takashi Kondo, and Takahisa Yamasaki

Abstract

There are various diagnostic tools for gastroesophageal reflux disease (GERD), such as GERD questionnaires, endoscopy, PPI tests, pH monitoring, and impedance testing. The role of endoscopy in the diagnosis of GERD may vary depending on the region. However, diagnosis of GERD should be based on symptoms, and these modalities should be used to assist in diagnosis. One should be aware not only of the diagnostic yield of these tests but also the physical and economic burden due to their use. This basic concept does not differ whether one is in Asia, the USA, or Europe. The diagnostic modalities for GERD continue to advance. Ideally, skillful combination of these new techniques with current practice will continue to bring improved therapeutic outcomes in GERD patients.

Keywords

PPI tests • pH monitoring • Quest • Frequency scale for the symptoms of GERD (FSSG) • Impedance test

Introduction

The prevalence of GERD in Asia has increased in recent years [1–3], and the method of diagnosis is becoming increasingly important. The diagnosis of GERD not only involves history-taking and symptom analysis but also gastrointestinal endoscopy and proton pump inhibitor (PPI) tests. Impedance tests and pH monitoring are conducted at specialized medical institutions. The fact that there are numerous

H. Miwa (✉) • T. Kondo • T. Yamasaki
Division of Gastroenterology, Department of Internal Medicine, Hyogo College of Medicine,
1-1, Mukogawa-cho, Nishinomiya, Hyogo, Japan, 663-8501
e-mail: miwahgi@hyo-med.ac.jp

© Springer India 2018

51

P. Sharma et al. (eds.), *The Rise of Acid Reflux in Asia*,
DOI 10.1007/978-81-322-0846-4_5

diagnostic modalities suggests that not only is the diagnosis difficult but also that one needs to understand the characteristics of the respective diagnostic modalities, as well as their advantages and disadvantages when diagnosing GERD. A good understanding of the best diagnostic tool in a given case is also important. This chapter will give an outline of the various diagnostic modalities for the diagnosis of GERD and also discuss which diagnostic tools are best suited for the same.

Issues and Controversies Surrounding Symptom-Based Diagnosis of GERD

The greatest problem for GERD patients is the marked decrease in quality of life (QOL) [4, 5]. The REQUEST study was done in a cohort of Japanese patients with reflux esophagitis and has shown a decrease in health-related quality of life (HRQOL) [6], which correlated with GERD symptoms. The purpose of GERD therapy is to alleviate symptoms and improve QOL and to enable the patient to lead a comfortable life. GERD treatment should be directed toward primarily reduction or disappearance of symptoms. In addition to being the most effective, a diagnosis based on symptoms is the most convenient and least invasive method. It is the most economical way to make a diagnosis. According to a large-scale questionnaire survey conducted among 847 gastrointestinal specialists in six East Asian countries, the tools used to diagnose GERD were symptoms in 61% of cases, endoscopy in 31%, PPI tests in 21%, a GERD-specific questionnaire in 10%, pH monitoring in 7%, and impedance testing in 3%. Symptoms were the most common basis for diagnosis [7].

However, individual patients may report the same symptoms differently, and these individual differences must be taken into consideration. For example, typical symptoms of GERD such as heartburn and acid reflux may be perceived differently between individuals, and not all patients will necessarily experience similar symptoms. In practice, heartburn may be understood differently by healthy subjects, patients with erosive or nonerosive esophagitis (NERD), and medical staff. In addition, these different groups may associate heartburn with a wide range of symptoms [8]. Furthermore, understanding of the symptom "heartburn" may differ based on race, sex, culture, and individual differences, and some authorities suggest that the understanding of heartburn symptoms may differ between Asia and Western countries [9]. A study in the USA investigated the frequency of heartburn and the level of understanding of the term "heartburn" in Caucasian, African-American, and Asian subjects; the results suggested that Asians report a low incidence of heartburn and have little understanding of that condition [10]. This suggests that symptom-based diagnosis of GERD might be less precise in that population. A modality to assist with or confirm GERD diagnosis is thus required.

The Utility of a Medical Questionnaire in GERD Diagnosis

Medical questionnaires are used in order to increase the effectiveness of diagnosis based on symptoms or to objectively assess therapeutic effects. These questionnaires may also be used to aid in the diagnosis of GERD by general practitioners. The self-administered medical questionnaire for diagnosis of reflux disease (QUEST) devised by Carlsson and Dent in 1998 is widely used [11]. It comprises seven items that are characteristic of GERD (presence of subjective symptoms associated with GERD including heartburn and chest pain, relationship to meals, relationship to meal contents, response to antacids, posture-based change in symptoms, effects of activities that increase intraabdominal pressure, change in symptoms when reflux occurs). When the cutoff score is set at four points, sensitivity is 70% and specificity is 46% for erosive GERD and 92% and 19%, respectively, for GERD.

The GERD Q is also a self-administered patient questionnaire; its usefulness was reported in 2009 during a large-scale clinical study in Europe (DIAMOND study) [12]. It has a total of six questions: three questions from the Reflux Disease Questionnaire (RDQ) [13], one question from the Gastrointestinal Symptom Rating Scale (GSRS) [14], and two questions from the Gastroesophageal Reflux Disease Impact Scale (GIS) [15]. The GERD Q has fewer question items than the QUEST questionnaire and was created to be a useful diagnostic tool in primary care. The sensitivity and specificity for GERD are 65% and 71%, respectively [12], making it non-inferior to the QUEST questionnaire. The score from the GERD Q questionnaire has been shown to correlate with reflux esophagitis at endoscopy and to the results of esophageal pH monitoring [12]. The usefulness of the GERD Q questionnaire has also been reported in a multicenter survey in China [16].

In Japan, the frequency scale for the symptom of GERD (FSSG), developed by Kusano et al. in 2004, is also used [17]. The FSSG consists of simple questions about the 12 highest-ranked symptoms that are commonly seen in GERD. These symptoms are ranked for frequency on a scale of 0–4. The higher the total score, the higher the possibility of GERD. When the cutoff value is set at eight points, the sensitivity is 75% and the specificity is 64%, i.e., similar to the QUEST questionnaire [18]. The FSSG is better suited than other questionnaires to assess improvement in therapeutic effects and is widely used in Japan.

In other parts of Asia, however, sensitivity and specificity are approximately 70%, regardless of which questionnaire is used. Since the level of understanding of symptoms like heartburn is lower than in Europe and America [9, 10], proposals have been made to use translations of foreign-language questionnaires into local languages or to develop original questionnaires in the non-English-speaking countries of Asia [19].

The PPI Test

If typical symptoms of GERD (heartburn and acid reflux or regurgitation) are present, then a PPI test may be used to confirm the diagnosis. The patient is given a high-dose PPI orally for 1–2 weeks; a positive therapeutic response indicates the presence of GERD. This test is conducted routinely in Western countries because it enables diagnosis of GERD noninvasively and is convenient and cheap [20]. When used only for diagnosis, the high-dose PPI is administered for 1–2 weeks; when used therapeutically, it is administered for 1–4 months [21]. In Western countries, the sensitivity and specificity of GERD diagnosis using the PPI test are 75%–90% and 45%–71%, respectively [22–27]. The test is considered useful for early-stage diagnosis. However, in East Asia, the method used for GERD diagnosis is largely dependent on the level of health care and medical economic conditions in each country. In countries like Japan and South Korea, endoscopy tends to be more commonly done than the PPI test to exclude GERD as a cause of symptoms [7]. The frequency of infection with *H. pylori* is higher in Asia than in Western countries, and there is a higher background morbidity of organic diseases such as gastric cancer and gastroduodenal ulcers. Thus, both doctors and patients tend to prefer an endoscopic examination as the first choice for diagnosis of GERD. This practice was supported in a recent report that checking for *H. pylori* and performing endoscopy are more cost-effective than the empirical PPI test in Asia, where the *H. pylori* infection rate is high [28]. On the other hand, physicians in the USA tend to be reluctant to use endoscopy as an early diagnostic option for GERD. The American College of Physicians (ACP) recommends the use of upper gastrointestinal endoscopy in patients who have warning symptoms (including dysphagia, bleeding, anemia, weight loss, recurrent vomiting) in addition to heartburn; also endoscopy should be done only if there is no success from a trial of PPI treatment lasting 4–8 weeks [29] and that unnecessary endoscopies should be avoided. This new way of thinking is also advocated in Asia, where endoscopy should be limited to high-risk groups such as elderly patients and those with dyspepsia, a history of ulcers, a family history of gastric cancer, or the presence of warning symptoms [30]. A multicenter study (the FUTURE study) was recently conducted in Japan on patients who presented with upper gastrointestinal symptoms including heartburn and were diagnosed with "chronic gastritis" by their physician. Gastric or esophageal cancer was noted in only 0.2% of those who underwent endoscopy, and organic disease was noted in only 6.2% [31]. In Asia, further data will be required to determine whether it is truly necessary to perform endoscopy before the PPI test.

According to the Montreal definition [9], "GERD is a condition that develops when the reflux of gastric content causes troublesome symptoms or complications," which includes extraesophageal symptoms as well as the typical symptoms. Among the extraesophageal symptoms, it is important to differentiate non-cardiac chest pain (NCCP) from conditions that require emergency management, such as acute coronary syndrome or dissecting aortic aneurysm. In a review of NCCP and GERD, Liuzzo et al. [32] reported that GERD was present in 44% of NCCP cases and that a direct relationship was found between chest pain and reflux in a high percentage of subjects (67%). There are also reports that 26–35% of asthma patients [33–35] and 75% of chronic cough patients [36] were found to have GERD. Thus, there is value in first attempting a PPI test in patients with suspected GERD due to atypical or extraesophageal symptoms without the typical symptoms of heartburn or acid reflux. Findings from a meta-analysis suggest that it is reasonable to use a PPI test to identify and diagnose GERD patients from among NCCP patients [37] and that NCCP patients can also experience therapeutic effects from PPIs [38]. The Asia Pacific Consensus on the management of GERD suggested that a therapeutic trial of PPI for patients with NCCP remains the most practical approach in primary care, owing to the low sensitivity of endoscopy and limited access to pH monitoring [39]. The PPI test is also reported to be useful for diagnosing asthma patients [40] and patients with laryngopharyngeal symptoms [41, 42].

GERD Diagnosis Using pH Monitoring

In a patient who does not respond to PPI, endoscopy should be performed. However, endoscopy is normal in about 71–95% of GERD patients from Asia [43]. In such patients, pH monitoring and impedance examinations may be required to investigate the relationship between acid reflux and the appearance of the symptoms. This procedure is useful for providing a definitive diagnosis in patients who complain about typical and/or atypical symptoms of GERD, regardless of whether there is obvious mucosal injury in the esophagus. Since pH monitoring can directly quantify the gastric acid reflux within the esophagus and can examine the relationship between the symptoms reported by the patient and actual reflux, it provides valuable information not available from other tests and procedures. Indices such as the symptom index (SI) [44, 45], symptom sensitivity index (SSI) [46], and symptom-association probability (SAP) [47] are used to assess the relationship between symptoms that occur during the investigation and actual reflux. Two US guidelines mention the indications for pH monitoring in clinical use [48, 49]. In Asia, the monitoring of pH is conducted primarily at research institutions.

In patients positive for GERD on endoscopy, reproducibility for two pH monitorings is 84–93% [50], and diagnostic sensitivity and specificity are reported to be 75%–96% and 60%–100%, respectively [51]. Monitoring of pH is thus considered an excellent method of detecting acid reflux within the esophagus. However, no abnormal acid reflux is noted in 50% of nonerosive reflux disease (NERD) patients, and of those, 63% are reported to have a symptom index below 50%. In NERD, patients with symptoms may often have no relationship to acid reflux [52]. In addition, conventional pH monitoring seen in PPI-resistant GERD patients shows normal values in 69% of patients receiving usual doses of PPI and in 96% of patients on double doses [53]. In other words, in NERD and PPI-resistant GERD, even if pH metry is normal, GERD symptoms may be present due to non-acid reflux or reflux of gas or gastric contents. Such conditions cannot be detected by pH monitoring. Conventional pH monitoring requires insertion of a transnasal pH catheter which restricts daily activities and causes mild discomfort to the patient. In order to resolve these problems, the pH measurement capsule, which is endoscopically attached to the esophageal mucosa, has been in use in the last few years; pH is monitored by a wireless device (Bravo-R) that permits evaluation for 24–48 h. These devices are being used in a clinical setting in Europe and the USA. However, the capsule is expensive, and occasionally the capsule may detach early (within 16 h in 3.5% of patients and within 36 h in 10.6%) [54].

Combined Multichannel Intraluminal Impedance and pH (MII-pH) Monitoring

Conventional esophageal pH monitoring has been limited to evaluation of pH changes within the esophagus (Figs. 5.1, 5.2, and 5.3). The esophageal impedance test can determine whether gastroesophageal reflux is due to antegrade or retrograde movement of the esophageal contents. It is also possible to assess the characteristics of reflux contents, i.e., whether they are liquid or gas or a combination of the two. Additionally, the most useful characteristic of the MII-pH method is the ability to simultaneously measure pH at multiple locations in the esophagus and thus to determine whether the refluxate is acidic or non-acidic [55]. The indications for impedance monitoring in the ACG guidelines [49] include the treatment of PPI-resistant NERD in patients who complain of heartburn and acid reflux after PPI treatment. According to Bredenoord et al., the indications for this modality include reflux symptoms resistant to inhibition of acid secretion, unexplained chronic cough, suspicion of rumination, excessive belching, and reflux symptoms in achlorhydria [56]. In 168 GERD patients who remained PPI resistant even after treatment with double-dose PPI, Vela et al. performed 24-h esophageal MII-pH monitoring while the patients were receiving PPI. Results showed that 16 patients (11%) had acid reflux associated with symptoms, and 53 patients (37%) had non-acid reflux with a positive symptom index. They also reported that, in PPI-resistant GERD, symptoms were caused by non-acid reflux in 37% of patients under treatment with PPIs [57]. It is possible that reflux in these patients gets overlooked during conventional pH monitoring. Such findings serve to highlight the usefulness of clinical application of

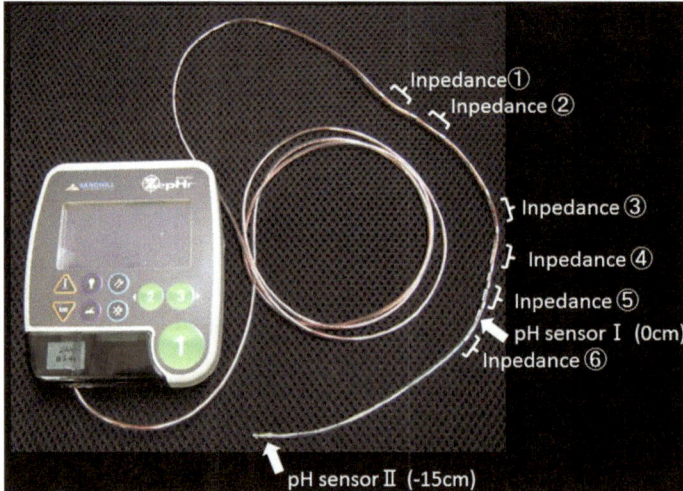

Fig. 5.1 *Impedance-pH monitoring.* We usually use this catheter which has ≥18-cm esophageal length, 6 impedance (spaced 2 cm), 2 pH channels (gastric and esophageal), −15 and 0 cm, diameter 6.4 FR/2.13 mm (ComforTec MII, Sandhill Scientific, Inc. Highland Ranch, CO, USA)

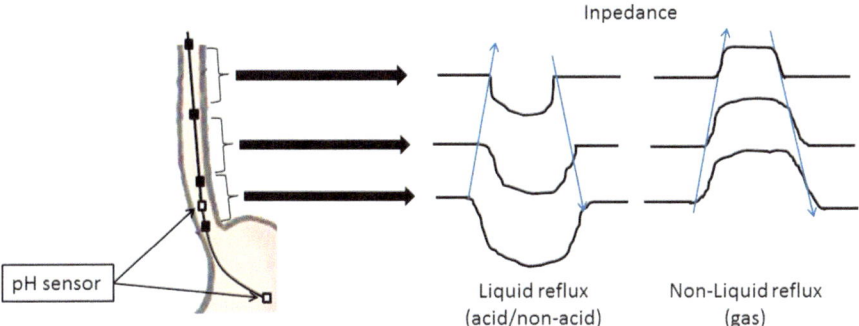

Fig. 5.2 *Schematic illustration for rationale of impedance.* In liquid reflux, the impedance decreases as the electric resistance of the catheter membrane decreases. In the reflux event, the impedance decreases sequentially from the lower part of the esophagus to the oral side. In the recovery phase, the impedance returns to the baseline from the oral to the lower part. A reflux episode was defined as the presence of a retrograde waveform showing a 50% decline in impedance from baseline. On the contrary, gas provides high electrical resistance which results in increment of the impedance. Also in gas reflux, the impedance increases from the lower part of the esophagus to the oral side and recovered in a reversed manner

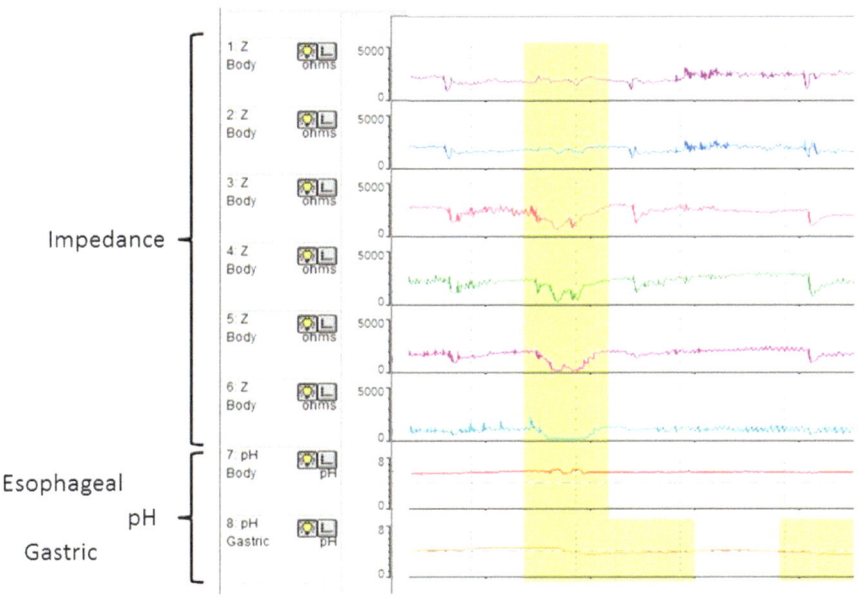

Fig. 5.3 *Presentation of the case with non-acid reflux detected by impedance-pH monitoring.* This is an impedance record showing the impedance-pH monitoring data of a 70-year-old woman with continuous epigastralgia. We see the reflux event that is shown in the yellow zone, where we notice the clearly decreased impedance waves on channel 3–6, suggesting this is a liquid reflux. At the same time, intraesophageal pH data on channel 7 did not show any pH changes, suggesting the reflux was non-acidic. We can also recognize the reflux liquid did not reach the upper part of the esophagus, as channels 1 and 2 did not detect impedance change

the impedance monitoring. In addition, the consensus regarding the definition and detection of acid reflux, non-acid reflux, and gas reflux during gastroesophageal reflux (GER) monitoring [58] indicates that an assessment of GERD by pH monitoring alone is insufficient. GERD symptoms are potentially associated with weakly acidic reflux and gas reflux that are not detected during pH monitoring, and that reflux is best detected using the MII-pH method. Patients in whom MII-pH monitoring does not show any evidence of reflux are likely to have functional heartburn or hypersensitivity of the esophagus [57, 59]. In other words, the MII-pH monitoring tests are able to capture acid/non-acid reflux in greater detail because the pH meter is combined with an impedance monitoring device. This makes it possible not only to detect pathology in PPI-resistant GERD and NERD patients but also to enable a new diagnostic classification of functional heartburn. Two impedance parameters evaluating esophageal chemical clearance (post-reflux swallow-induced peristaltic wave [PSPW] index) [60] and mucosal integrity (mean nocturnal baseline impedance [MNBI]) [61] are under evaluation. The PSPW index [60] assesses chemical clearance after an episode of reflux; lower values are found in erosive reflux disease (ERD) than in nonerosive reflux disease (NERD). MNBI helps to distinguish hypersensitive esophagus from functional heartburn [61]. Recently, Frazzoni et al. concluded that the PSPW index and MNBI increase the diagnostic yield of impedance pH monitoring in patients with reflux disease, as compared with pH-only data [62].

Conclusions

The basis of GERD therapy is a diagnosis based on symptoms; various diagnostic tools such as GERD questionnaires, endoscopy findings, PPI tests, pH monitoring, and impedance tests are used to support and verify this symptom-based diagnosis. The diagnostic modalities for GERD continue to advance. However, unless a diagnosis is based on symptoms, we should be aware that the physical and economic burden of the tests placed on patients is considerable. These modalities should be used to assist in diagnosis, rather than play a central role. This basic concept does not differ, whether one is in Asia or in the USA or Europe. Ideally, skillful combination of these new techniques with current practice will continue to bring improved therapeutic outcomes for GERD patients.

References

1. Fujiwara Y, Arakawa T. Epidemiology and clinical characteristics of GERD in the Japanese population. J Gastroenterol. 2009;44:518–34.
2. Ho KY. From GERD to Barrett's esophagus: is the pattern in Asia mirroring that in the West? J Gastroenterol Hepatol. 2011;26:816–24.
3. Jung HK. Epidemiology of gastroesophageal reflux disease in Asia: a systematic review. J Neurogastroenterol Motil. 2011;17:14–27.
4. Dimenas E. Methodological aspects of evaluation of quality of life in upper gastrointestinal diseases. Scand J Gastroenterol Suppl. 1993;199:18–21.

5. Wiklund I. Quality of life in patients with gastroesophageal reflux disease. Am J Gastroenterol. 2001;96:S46–53.
6. Hongo M, Kinoshita Y, Miwa H, Ashida K. The demographic characteristics and health-related quality of life in a large cohort of reflux esophagitis patients in Japan with reference to the effect of lansoprazole: the REQUEST study. J Gastroenterol. 2008;43:920–7.
7. Fujiwara Y, Takahashi S, Arakawa T, Sollano JD, Zhu Q, Kachintorn U, et al. A 2008 questionnaire-based survey of gastroesophageal reflux disease and related diseases by physicians in East Asian countries. Digestion. 2009;80:119–28.
8. Manabe N, Haruma K, Hata J, Kamada T, Kusunoki H. Differences in recognition of heartburn symptoms between Japanese patients with gastroesophageal reflux, physicians, nurses, and healthy lay subjects. Scand J Gastroenterol. 2008;43:398–402.
9. Vakil N, van Zanten SV, Kahrilas P, Dent J, Jones R. The Montreal definition and classification of gastroesophageal reflux disease: a global evidence-based consensus. Am J Gastroenterol. 2006;101:1900–20. quiz 1943
10. Spechler SJ, Jain SK, Tendler DA, Parker RA. Racial differences in the frequency of symptoms and complications of gastro-oesophageal reflux disease. Aliment Pharmacol Ther. 2002;16:1795–800.
11. Carlsson R, Dent J, Bolling-Sternevald E, Johnsson F, Junghard O, Lauritsen K, et al. The usefulness of a structured questionnaire in the assessment of symptomatic gastroesophageal reflux disease. Scand J Gastroenterol. 1998;33:1023–9.
12. Jones R, Junghard O, Dent J, Vakil N, Halling K, Wernersson B, et al. Development of the GerdQ, a tool for the diagnosis and management of gastro-oesophageal reflux disease in primary care. Aliment Pharmacol Ther. 2009;30:1030–8.
13. Shaw M, Dent J, Beebe T, Junghard O, Wiklund I, Lind T, et al. The reflux disease questionnaire: a measure for assessment of treatment response in clinical trials. Health Qual Life Outcomes. 2008;6:31.
14. Revicki DA, Wood M, Wiklund I, Crawley J. Reliability and validity of the gastrointestinal symptom rating scale in patients with gastroesophageal reflux disease. Qual Life Res. 1998;7:75–83.
15. Jones R, Coyne K, Wiklund I. The gastro-oesophageal reflux disease impact scale: a patient management tool for primary care. Aliment Pharmacol Ther. 2007;25:1451–9.
16. Bai Y, Du Y, Zou D, Jin Z, Zhan X, Li ZS, et al. Gastroesophageal reflux disease questionnaire (GerdQ) in real-world practice: a national multicenter survey on 8065 patients. J Gastroenterol Hepatol. 2013;28:626–31.
17. Kusano M, Shimoyama Y, Sugimoto S, Kawamura O, Maeda M, Minashi K, et al. Development and evaluation of FSSG: frequency scale for the symptoms of GERD. J Gastroenterol. 2004;39:888–91.
18. Nonaka T, Kessoku T, Ogawa Y, Yanagisawa S, Shiba T, Sakaguchi T, et al. Comparative study of 2 different questionnaires in Japanese patients: the quality of life and utility evaluation survey technology questionnaire (QUEST) versus the frequency scale for the symptoms of Gastroesophageal reflux disease questionnaire (FSSG). J Neurogastroenterol Motil. 2013;19:54–60.
19. Fock KM, Talley NJ, Fass R, Goh KL, Katelaris P, Hunt R, et al. Asia-Pacific consensus on the management of gastroesophageal reflux disease: update. J Gastroenterol Hepatol. 2008;23:8–22.
20. Gasiorowska A, Fass R. The proton pump inhibitor (PPI) test in GERD: does it still have a role? J Clin Gastroenterol. 2008;42:867–74.
21. Dekel R, Morse C, Fass R. The role of proton pump inhibitors in gastro-oesophageal reflux disease. Drugs. 2004;64:277–95.
22. Johnsson F, Weywadt L, Solhaug JH, Hernqvist H, Bengtsson L. One-week omeprazole treatment in the diagnosis of gastro-oesophageal reflux disease. Scand J Gastroenterol. 1998;33:15–20.

23. Fass R, Fennerty MB, Ofman JJ, Gralnek IM, Johnson C, Camargo E, et al. The clinical and economic value of a short course of omeprazole in patients with noncardiac chest pain. Gastroenterology. 1998;115:42–9.
24. Juul-Hansen P, Rydning A, Jacobsen CD, Hansen T. High-dose proton-pump inhibitors as a diagnostic test of gastro-oesophageal reflux disease in endoscopic-negative patients. Scand J Gastroenterol. 2001;36:806–10.
25. des Varannes SB, Sacher-Huvelin S, Vavasseur F, Masliah C, Le Rhun M, Aygalenq P, et al. Rabeprazole test for the diagnosis of gastro-oesophageal reflux disease: results of a study in a primary care setting. World J Gastroenterol. 2006;12:2569–73.
26. Tseng PH, Lee YC, Chiu HM, Wang HP, Lin JT, Wu MS. A comparative study of proton-pump inhibitor tests for Chinese reflux patients in relation to the CYP2C19 genotypes. J Clin Gastroenterol. 2009;43:920–5.
27. Lee YC, Lin JT, Wang HP, Chiu HM, Wu MS. Influence of cytochrome P450 2C19 genetic poly-morphism and dosage of rabeprazole on accuracy of proton-pump inhibitor testing in Chinese patients with gastroesophageal reflux disease. J Gastroenterol Hepatol. 2007;22:1286–92.
28. You JH, Wong PL, Wu JC. Cost-effectiveness of helicobacter pylori "test and treat" for patients with typical reflux symptoms in a population with a high prevalence of H. pylori infection: a Markov model analysis. Scand J Gastroenterol. 2006;41:21–9.
29. Shaheen NJ, Weinberg DS, Denberg TD, Chou R, Qaseem A, Shekelle P. Upper endoscopy for gastroesophageal reflux disease: best practice advice from the clinical guidelines committee of the American College of Physicians. Ann Intern Med. 2012;157:808–16.
30. Wu JC. Gastroesophageal reflux disease: an Asian perspective. J Gastroenterol Hepatol. 2008;23:1785–93.
31. Kinoshita Y, Chiba T. Characteristics of Japanese patients with chronic gastritis and compari-son with functional dyspepsia defined by ROME III criteria: based on the large-scale survey. FUTURE study Intern Med. 2011;50:2269–76.
32. Liuzzo JP, Ambrose JA. Chest pain from gastroesophageal reflux disease in patients with coro-nary artery disease. Cardiol Rev. 2005;13:167–73.
33. Larrain A, Carrasco E, Galleguillos F, Sepulveda R, Pope CE 2nd. Medical and surgical treat-ment of nonallergic asthma associated with gastroesophageal reflux. Chest. 1991;99:1330–5.
34. Kiljander TO, Salomaa ER, Hietanen EK, Terho EO. Gastroesophageal reflux in asthmatics: a double-blind, placebo-controlled crossover study with omeprazole. Chest. 1999;116:1257–64.
35. Irwin RS, Curley FJ, French CL. Difficult-to-control asthma. Contributing factors and out-come of a systematic management protocol. Chest. 1993;103:1662–9.
36. Irwin RS, French CL, Curley FJ, Zawacki JK, Bennett FM. Chronic cough due to gastro-esophageal reflux. Clinical, diagnostic, and pathogenetic aspects. Chest. 1993;104:1511–7.
37. Wang WH, Huang JQ, Zheng GF, Wong WM, Lam SK, Karlberg J, et al. Is proton pump inhibitor testing an effective approach to diagnose gastroesophageal reflux disease in patients with noncardiac chest pain?: a meta-analysis. Arch Intern Med. 2005;165:1222–8.
38. Cremonini F, Wise J, Moayyedi P, Talley NJ. Diagnostic and therapeutic use of proton pump inhibitors in non-cardiac chest pain: a metaanalysis. Am J Gastroenterol. 2005;100:1226–32.
39. Fock KM, Talley N, Goh KL, Sugano K, Katelaris P, Holtmann G, et al. Asia-Pacific consensus on the management of gastro-oesophageal reflux disease: an update focusing on refractory reflux disease and Barrett's oesophagus. Gut. 2016;65:1402–15.
40. Field SK, Sutherland LR. Does medical antireflux therapy improve asthma in asthmatics with gastroesophageal reflux?: a critical review of the literature. Chest. 1998;114:275–83.
41. Kamel PL, Hanson D, Kahrilas PJ. Omeprazole for the treatment of posterior laryngitis. Am J Med. 1994;96:321–6.
42. Wo JM, Grist WJ, Gussack G, Delgaudio JM, Waring JP. Empiric trial of high-dose omeprazole in patients with posterior laryngitis: a prospective study. Am J Gastroenterol. 1997;92:2160–5.
43. Goh KL. Gastroesophageal reflux disease in Asia: a historical perspective and present chal-lenges. J Gastroenterol Hepatol. 2011;26(Suppl 1):2–10.

44. Wiener GJ, Richter JE, Copper JB, Wu WC, Castell DO. The symptom index: a clinically important parameter of ambulatory 24-hour esophageal pH monitoring. Am J Gastroenterol. 1988;83:358–61.
45. Singh S, Richter JE, Bradley LA, Haile JM. The symptom index. Differential usefulness in suspected acid-related complaints of heartburn and chest pain. Dig Dis Sci. 1993;38:1402–8.
46. Breumelhof R, Smout AJ. The symptom sensitivity index: a valuable additional parameter in 24-hour esophageal pH recording. Am J Gastroenterol. 1991;86:160–4.
47. Weusten BL, Roelofs JM, Akkermans LM, Van Berge-Henegouwen GP, Smout AJ. The symptom-association probability: an improved method for symptom analysis of 24-hour esophageal pH data. Gastroenterology. 1994;107:1741–5.
48. Kahrilas PJ, Quigley EM. Clinical esophageal pH recording: a technical review for practice guideline development. Gastroenterology. 1996;110:1982–96.
49. Hirano I, Richter JE. ACG practice guidelines: esophageal reflux testing. Am J Gastroenterol. 2007;102:668–85.
50. Wiener GJ, Morgan TM, Copper JB, Wu WC, Castell DO, Sinclair JW, et al. Ambulatory 24-hour esophageal pH monitoring. Reproducibility and variability of pH parameters. Dig Dis Sci. 1988;33:1127–33.
51. Klinkenberg-Knol EC, Meuwissen SG. Combined gastric and oesophageal 24-hour pH monitoring and oesophageal manometry in patients with reflux disease, resistant to treatment with omeprazole. Aliment Pharmacol Ther. 1990;4:485–95.
52. Martinez SD, Malagon IB, Garewal HS, Cui H, Fass R. Non-erosive reflux disease (NERD)--acid reflux and symptom patterns. Aliment Pharmacol Ther. 2003;17:537–45.
53. Charbel S, Khandwala F, Vaezi MF. The role of esophageal pH monitoring in symptomatic patients on PPI therapy. Am J Gastroenterol. 2005;100:283–9.
54. Pandolfino JE, Richter JE, Ours T, Guardino JM, Chapman J, Kahrilas PJ. Ambulatory esophageal pH monitoring using a wireless system. Am J Gastroenterol. 2003;98:740–9.
55. Tutuian R, Castell DO. Review article: complete gastro-oesophageal reflux monitoring - combined pH and impedance. Aliment Pharmacol Ther. 2006;24(Suppl 2):27–37.
56. Bredenoord AJ, Tutuian R, Smout AJ, Castell DO. Technology review: esophageal impedance monitoring. Am J Gastroenterol. 2007;102:187–94.
57. Vela MF. Non-acid reflux: detection by multichannel intraluminal impedance and pH, clinical significance and management. Am J Gastroenterol. 2009;104:277–80.
58. Sifrim D, Castell D, Dent J, Kahrilas PJ. Gastro-oesophageal reflux monitoring: review and consensus report on detection and definitions of acid, non-acid, and gas reflux. Gut. 2004;53:1024–31.
59. Savarino E, Zentilin P, Tutuian R, Pohl D, Casa DD, Frazzoni M, et al. The role of nonacid reflux in NERD: lessons learned from impedance-pH monitoring in 150 patients off therapy. Am J Gastroenterol. 2008;103:2685–93.
60. Frazzoni M, Manta R, Mirante VG, Conigliaro R, Frazzoni L, Melotti G. Esophageal chemical clearance is impaired in gastro-esophageal reflux disease--a 24-h impedance-pH monitoring assessment. Neurogastroenterol Motil. 2013;25:399–406.
61. Martinucci I, De Bortoli N, Savarino E, Piaggi P, Bellini M, Antonelli A, et al. Esophageal baseline impedance levels in patients with pathophysiological characteristics of functional heartburn. Neurogastroenterol Motil. 2014;26:546–55.
62. Frazzoni M, Savarino E, de Bortoli N, Martinucci I, Furnari M, Frazzoni M, et al. Analyses of the post-reflux swallow-induced peristaltic wave index and nocturnal baseline impedance parameters increase the diagnostic yield of impedance-pH monitoring of patients with reflux disease. Clin Gastroenterol Hepatol. 2016;14:40–6.

Role of Endoscopy and Novel Imaging in GERD

6

Rupa Banerjee and Duvvur Nageshwar Reddy

Introduction

Gastro esophageal reflux disease (GERD) is a condition which develops due to reflux of gastric contents into the esophagus causing symptoms, complications, or both.

GERD-related symptoms are common, affecting 25–30% of the general population in the west. Recent studies suggest a worldwide increase in prevalence of at least 4% per year [1].

GERD is less prevalent in the Asia Pacific region but appears to be on a rapidly rising phase [2]. Needless to say, it causes a significant decrease in quality of life and is a huge economic burden [3, 4].

Upper gastrointestinal endoscopy and examination of the esophagus has been the most widely used modality for the diagnosis and grading of severity of erosive reflux disease and its complications. It also allows tissue sampling and application of therapeutic procedures like dilatation and endoscopic mucosal resection [5]. Quite expectedly, with the increasing prevalence of GERD, the usage of upper GI endoscopy is on the rise.

Standard endoscopy using white light endoscopy has been the norm. However, more than 60% of patients with reflux symptoms suffer from nonerosive reflux disease (NERD) and show no visible changes on white light endoscopy (WLE).

Novel imaging technologies are now evolving which enable better visualization of mucosal details. These technological advances, such as digital chromoendoscopy, help circumvent the limitations of WLE in reflux disease by (a) improved detection of subtle irregularities and (b) characterization of anomalies and possible optical biopsies, providing real-time diagnosis.

R. Banerjee (✉) • D.N. Reddy
Asian Institute of Gastroenterology, Hyderabad, India
e-mail: aigindia@yahoo.co.in

© Springer India 2018
P. Sharma et al. (eds.), *The Rise of Acid Reflux in Asia*,
DOI 10.1007/978-81-322-0846-4_6

This chapter aims to discuss the role and appropriate utilization of endoscopy and novel imaging technology in patients with GERD.

Indications for Endoscopy in GERD

High-definition, high-resolution endoscopy is now widely available and accepted as standard endoscopic care for GERD across the globe. It enables direct visualization of the esophageal and gastric mucosa and allows tissue sampling for histology. GERD is the most common indication for endoscopy.

It is important to clarify here that the diagnosis of GERD can usually be made on the basis of clinical symptoms alone. Additionally, as mentioned earlier, 50–85% of patients with GERD have nonerosive reflux disease with a normal endoscopy. The sensitivity of endoscopy for GERD is low, but it has high specificity at 90–95%. Empiric medical therapy with once-daily proton pump inhibitors is therefore an appropriate initial step for uncomplicated disease, and a routine endoscopy is not warranted. Endoscopy is indicated only if 4–8 weeks of twice-daily PPI fails to resolve the symptoms [6].

It has been debated whether a screening endoscopy should be done in patients with well-controlled symptoms for detection of complications like Barrett's esophagus (BE) or esophageal adenocarcinoma. However, an endoscopy in every patient with GERD would be a low-yield, high-cost procedure and would still not detect BE in asymptomatic individuals. Also, numerous studies have now shown that the absolute risk of adenocarcinoma in women even with symptoms is low. Similarly, the incidence is low in patients <50 years of age and the non-Caucasian population. Recent guidelines by the British Society of Gastroenterology have clearly stated that screening endoscopy in an unselected population with reflux symptoms is not feasible [7]. A reasonable and plausible approach would be to individualize to patients with chronic symptoms with multiple risk factors (at least three of: age 50 years or older, white race, male sex, obesity). A family history of adenocarcinoma would also warrant an early examination.

Endoscopy at presentation is indicated only in certain specific situations, listed below. These include the presence of alarm symptoms of weight loss, dysphagia, anemia, bleeding, or recurrent vomiting, or the presence of extra-esophageal symptoms like hoarseness of voice and cough. The probability of lesion detection is much higher in the presence of alarm symptoms. In a recent retrospective analysis of 30,337 patients with dysphagia as an alarm symptom, more than 50% had significant findings, primarily stricture formation.

Indications for Endoscopy in Patients with GERD

1. GERD symptoms that are persistent or progressive despite appropriate medical therapy
2. Dysphagia or odynophagia
3. Involuntary weight loss O5%

4. Evidence of GI bleeding or anemia
5. Finding of a mass, stricture, or ulcer on imaging studies
6. Evaluation of patients with suspected extra-esophageal manifestations of GERD
7. Screening for BE in selected patients (as clinically indicated)
8. Persistent vomiting
9. Evaluation of patients with recurrent symptoms after endoscopic or surgical anti-reflux procedures

Follow-up endoscopy is advocated in patients with a documented severe esophagitis (Los Angeles classification: Grade B and above; Table 6.1) after 8 weeks of PPI therapy. This helps ensure complete healing and duration of PPI usage. Additionally, it can detect Barrett's esophagus in previously denuded esophageal epithelium. Generally, no further endoscopy is needed if the follow-up endoscopy is normal.

Repeated endoscopies are often needed in cases of esophageal strictures because recurrence is common, requiring repeated dilatations. The timing of these endoscopies can usually be guided by the presence and severity of symptoms. In asymptomatic patients with a history of a peptic stricture a repeat endoscopy is not required.

Table 6.1 The modified Los Angeles classification of esophagitis

Grades		Image
Grade A	One (or more) mucosal breaks no longer than 5 mm that do not extend between the tops of two mucosal folds	
Grade B	One (or more) mucosal break more than 5 mm long that do not extend between the tops of two mucosal folds	
Grade C	One (or more) mucosal breaks that are continuous between the tops of two or more mucosal folds but which involve less than 75% of the circumference	
Grade D	One (or more) mucosal breaks which involve at least 75% of the esophageal circumference	

Surveillance endoscopy has been advocated for the early detection of dysplasia and/or malignancy in BE by many guidelines. These have been based primarily on observational data studies that indicate that surveillance correlates with earlier stage and improved survival from cancer. There are no randomized controlled trials. Accordingly, upper endoscopy with multiple four-quadrant biopsies every 3 to 5 years is considered adequate. More frequent examinations may be required in patients with dysplasia due to the enhanced risk of progression. Serial endoscopy for the detection of BE in patients with chronic GERD symptoms is not recommended.

Endoscopy for Diagnosis and Grading of Severity of GERD

Upper endoscopy is the standard for documenting the presence and extent of esophagitis and excluding other etiologies for the patient's symptoms.

Edema and erythema are the earliest endoscopic signs of acid reflux, but these findings are nonspecific and dependent on the quality of endoscopic images. Other signs are friability, granularity, and red streaks as a direct consequence of gastric acid injury. Mucosal friability is due to enlarged capillaries near the mucosal surface. Red streaks develop upward along the ridges of the esophageal folds. Progressive acid injury causes shallow breaks or erosions in the mucosa surrounded by erythema.

Erosions start at the gastroesophageal junction, occurring along the tops of esophageal mucosal folds where acid injury is most prone. Finally, ulcers develop, indicating more severe form of esophageal damage involving mucosa or submucosa [8, 9].

Endoscopy also allows for biopsies in patients with irregular or deep ulceration and any mass lesion or obvious nodularity and to rule out Barrett's esophagus.

Numerous studies have shown a specificity of more than 95% for the diagnosis of GERD. However, it is important to remember here that more than 50% of patients with GERD symptoms have a normal endoscopy. Also, there is often no correlation between the severity of symptoms and the endoscopic findings. Empirical treatment with proton pump inhibitors resolves the symptoms in many cases, further supporting the recommendation that endoscopy is not warranted in all cases of GERD.

There are several classification systems for the grading of endoscopic severity of GERD. The Los Angeles (LA) classification has been the most widely used (see Table 6.1). The severity of endoscopic findings on LA classification has correlated well with the pH-metry data. This system has demonstrated good intra- and interobserver agreement [10].

Role of Newer Imaging Technologies in GERD and Complications

There are two primary limitations of conventional white light endoscopy (WLE) in the GERD spectrum:

Nonerosive Reflux Disease More than 60% of patients suffering from reflux symptoms show no visible changes on WLE [11]. Consequently, NERD has remained a heterogeneous disease with reflux symptoms and an unpredictable response to antireflux therapy. It appears possible that minute mucosal changes and minimal change esophagitis are not adequately visualized by conventional WLE [12, 13].

Barrett's Esophagus (BE) and Surveillance Amidst the increasing worldwide prevalence of GERD is the rising incidence of complications, including BE and esophageal adenocarcinoma [14]. Here again early neoplastic lesions are difficult to diagnose with WLE. Four-quadrant biopsies every 2 cm length is time consuming and has been associated with high sampling error. Moreover, the low incidence (0.5% per year) reduces the cost-effectiveness of this laborious surveillance measure (Fig. 6.1a and b) [14–16].

Endoscopic imaging today has evolved beyond the confines of white light endoscopy to advanced optical imaging with a precise and real-time endoscopic diagnosis [17]. It has also helped in the early diagnosis of complications with targeted biopsies (Fig. 6.2a and b).

These technological advances have helped circumvent the limitation of WLE in reflux disease by (a) improved detection of subtle irregularities, and (b) characterization of anomalies and possible optical biopsies, providing real-time diagnosis.

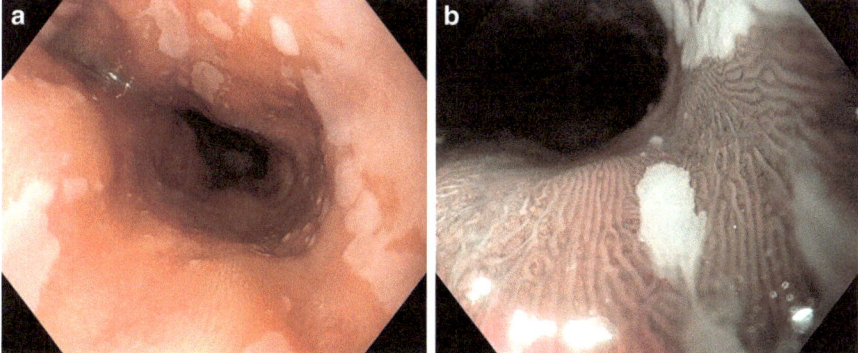

Fig. 6.1 (**a**) Barrett's esophagus on WLE; (**b**) on NBI a ridged pit pattern with regular vascular pattern clearly identified

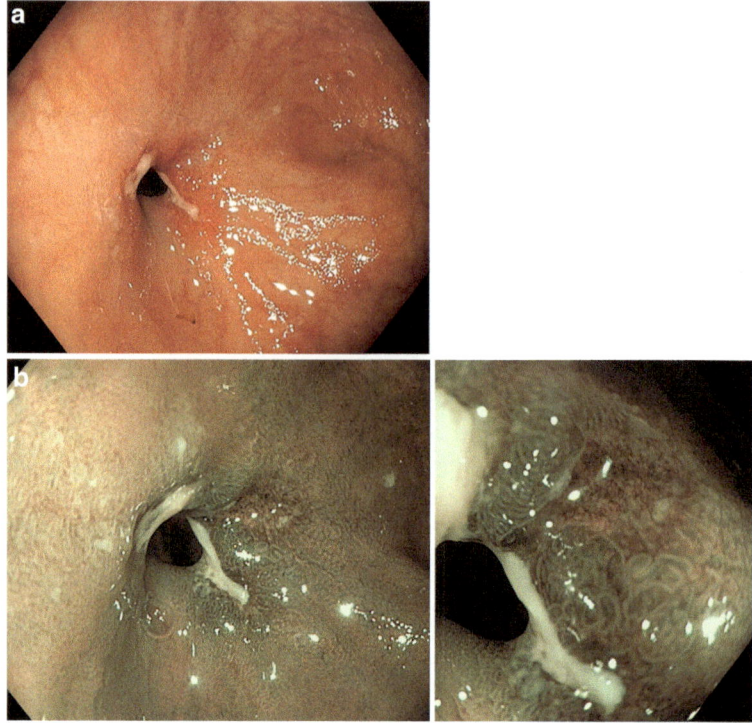

Fig. 6.2 NBI in the detection of complications. (**a**) Long-term peptic stricture with proximal ulceration on WLE. (**b**) Area of irregular microvessel pattern noted on NBI with magnification (inset). Carcinoma in situ detected on targeted biopsy

Newer imaging technologies used in GERD can be categorized into:

1. *Image-enhanced endoscopy or field enhancement* technologies. This involves contrast enhancement using dye (chromoendoscopy) or digital techniques including:
   (a) HRME
   (b) NBI, i-scan, FICE
   (c) Autofluorescence endoscopy
2. *Virtual histology or point enhancement* for in vivo histological examination during endoscopy:
   (a) Confocal laser endomicroscopy
   (b) Endocytoscopy

High-Resolution Magnification Endoscopy (HRME)

High-resolution magnification endoscopy (HRME) involves the use of high-resolution endoscopes of around 850 K pixel density with a movable lens and optical zooming facility of up to ×200 magnification. This results in a higher-resolution magnified image with the ability to detect and discriminate minute lesions [18].

HRME has been able to identify subtle changes such as punctuate erythema, pinpoint vessels, and triangular indentations above the Z line (GE junction) in subjects with otherwise normal WLE [12].

A few studies have evaluated these changes as markers of minimal change esophagitis in NERD. Kiesslich et al. demonstrated endoscopic signs of minimal change esophagitis for the prediction of NERD in 39 patients before and after treatment with esomeprazole [19]. In a small pilot study of 18 patients, we found subtle vascular pattern changes including the comma-shaped intrapapillary capillary loops in subjects with nonerosive reflux disease, which resolved after PPI therapy [20].

HRME was described for detection of BE by Guelrud in 2001 [21] and a Japanese group in 2002 [22]. Subsequently HRME alone for the characterization of BE has not been much reported. However, increased detection rates of intestinal dysplasia and high-grade dysplasia have been reported when HRME is used in conjunction with indigo carmine dye spraying or NBI [23].

The primary limitation of magnification endoscopy has been a substantial inter- and intraobserver variability with unacceptable kappa levels. The advent of newer generation endoscopes including narrow-band imaging with greater contrast enhancement has better defined and categorized the changes of both minimal change esophagitis and BE.

Chromoendoscopy

Chromoendoscopy involves the topical application of dyes for image enhancement during endoscopy. Vital stains which actively stain the cells and contrast stains, which are not absorbed but pool in the crevasses of the mucosa, are used. Of these, Lugol's iodine, methylene blue, and indigo carmine are most commonly used for the esophagus [18].

Lugol's iodine has been used to identify minimal mucosal breaks and can identify minimal change esophagitis in a subset of patients with NERD and normal WLE. Iodine is absorbed by the glycogen-containing nonkeratinized squamous epithelium of the normal esophagus. Inflammatory or dysplastic squamous epitheliums do not stain and appear as unstained streaks [24].

Methylene blue and indigo carmine spraying has primarily been used to characterize BE [25, 26]. Five distinct patterns of columnar-appearing mucosa have been identified including small/round, straight, long oval, tubular, and villous. Metaplastic tissue has been associated with the tubular and villous patterns in reported series. The results of chromoendoscopy for the diagnosis of dysplasia in BE have been quite inconsistent. However, there has been a consistent and significant reduction in the number of biopsies required for diagnosis [18, 26].

Overall chromoendoscopy has limited usage in GERD in view of inconsistent results, possible DNA effects of the vital dyes, inability to detect superficial vascular patterns, and of course the time-consuming and messy procedure. The advent of the no-dye "switch of the button" digital chromoendoscopy is set to replace chromoendoscopy [27–29].

Digital Chromoendoscopy (NBI/i-scan/FICE)

Digital chromoendoscopy has been developed as an alternative method of visual enhancement similar to chromoendoscopy. These novel optical technologies include narrow-band imaging (NBI), i-scan, and FICE, which can demonstrate and distinguish the alteration in the pit pattern and vasculature between inflammatory and neoplastic lesions [30].

Narrow-band imaging developed by Olympus Medical Systems (Olympus, Japan) is the most well-recognized advance in endoscopic imaging. This involves the placement of narrow-band pass filters to obtain tissue illumination at selected narrow wavelength bands, enhancing visualization and assisting in tissue characterization, differentiation, and diagnosis.

i-scan from Pentax (Montvale, NJ) and Fuji Intelligent Chromo Endoscopy (FICE) (Fujinon, Wayne, NJ) on the other hand involve spectral estimation technology and are based on post-imaging processing. There is no optical filter involved in contrast to NBI. Only a limited number of studies have been reported with i-scan/FICE.

NBI of the Normal Esophagus

On NBI, the stratified squamous epithelium of the esophagus appears featureless and has no pit pattern. There is a regular palisading capillary network. The intrapapillary capillary loop (IPCL) pattern, which is barely visible on WLE, is clearly outlined on NBI and plays an important role in the diagnosis of GERD and related complications [30]. The normal IPCL is a smooth-running, small-diameter capillary vessel positioned upright from a branching vessel about 10 μm in size. The branching vessels appear green, while the IPCLs are observed as dark brown loops/dots on NBI [31].

IPCLs have shown characteristic changes including dilatation, prolongation, meandering, and irregularity in form and caliber, according to the extent of tissue atypism from inflammation to dysplasia and cancer. Many of these publications are in Japanese. Inoue et al. have actually classified IPCLs from Type I (normal), Type II (inflammation), Type III (borderline), Type IV (carcinoma in situ), to Type V (invasive CA) (Fig. 6.3) [31, 32].

NBI Endoscopy in GERD

Conventional WLE has often been considered to be a relatively insensitive test for GERD because it is able to identify lesions in only 40% of cases with symptoms. [33] The ability of NBI to depict subtle mucosal lesions has improved the diagnostic accuracy in GERD.

Various subtle changes not seen regularly on WLE have been noted on NBI. These have included: (a) increased Type II IPCLs (elongated and arranged in linear orientation) above the Z line; (b) punctate erythema proximal to the Z line; (c) increased vascular markings distal to the Z line; (d) triangular indentations of columnar mucosa at the SC junction; and (e) islands of squamous epithelium distal to the Z line.

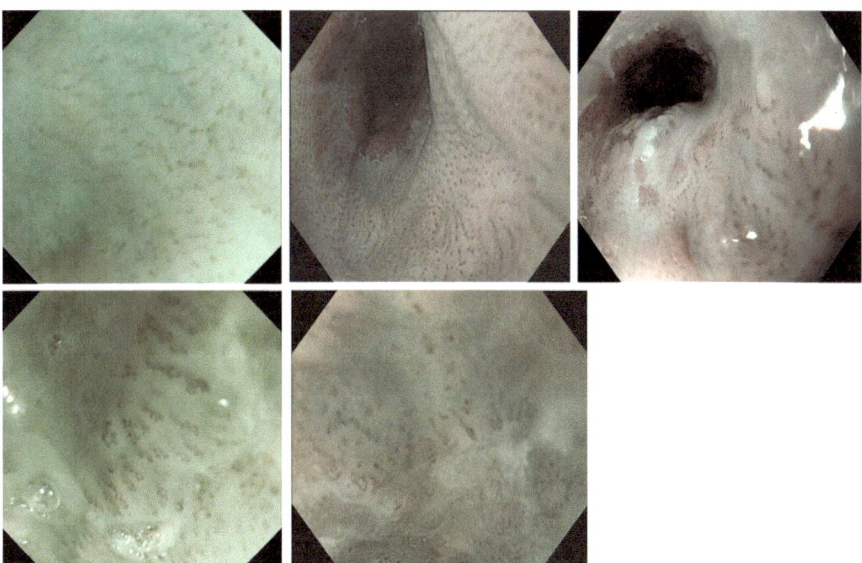

Fig. 6.3 The IPCLs: Type I to Type V. Note the gradual dilatation, tortuosity, and change in caliber from normal to esophageal malignancy

Some of these changes have been found to be reversible on PPI therapy and may represent the true endoscopic markers of minimal change esophagitis.

Sharma et al. in the landmark study of 80 patients with GERD reported an increased number and dilatation of IPCLs as the best predictors of GERD on multivariate analysis. The maximum, minimum, and average number of IPCLs per field was significantly greater in GERD. Also, a significantly higher proportion of patients with GERD had changes in the number (OR 12.6; $p > 0.00001$), dilatation (OR 20; $p > 0.0001$), and tortuosity (OR6.9; $p > 0.001$) of IPCLs [34].

Similarly, we evaluated 60 patients with NERD on WLE by NBI. Minimal changes were detected in 21 patients. Increased and dilated IPCLs were noted most frequently in 19/21 (90.4%) patients. Increased vascular markings with hyperemia and punctate erythema proximal to the Z line was detected in 15/21 (71.4%). Interestingly, these resolved in 95% cases on PPI (pantoprazole) therapy [35].

Fock et al. in a recent study of 107 subjects used simpler criteria to identify minimal change disease. Micro-erosions, increased vascularity, and pit pattern at the GE junction not seen on WLE were identified on NBI. Micro-erosions were present in 100%, 92.8%, and 23.3% of GERD, NERD, and controls, respectively. An increase in vascularity was noted in 95.1% GERD, 91.7% NERD, and 36.7% of controls. The increase in vascularity with the absence of round pit pattern was helpful to differentiate NERD from controls, with a sensitivity of 86.1% and specificity of 83.3%, respectively. In addition, there was good interobserver agreement for the presence of micro-erosions (kappa 0.89), increased vascularity at SCJ (kappa 0.95), and round pit pattern (kappa 0.80) [36].

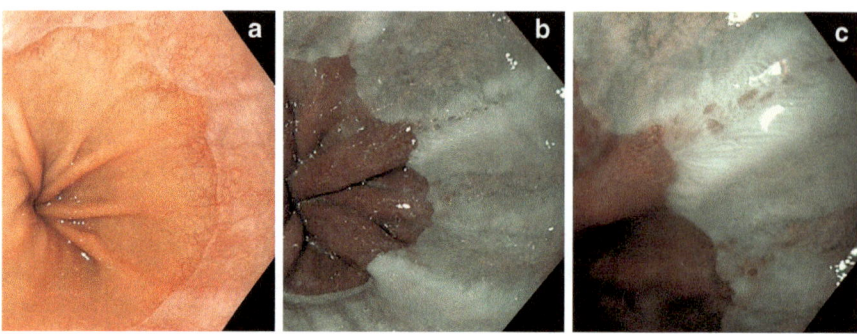

Figs 6.4 (**a**) Normal-appearing GE junction on WLE; (**b**) fine linear erosion clearly visible on NBI; (**c**) typical appearance of minimal change esophagitis with dilated IPCLs arranged in a linear fashion (inverted fir tree)

A recent study found subjects with minimal changes on NBI (normal on WLE) responded better to PPI. Accordingly, NBI could be used for prediction of therapeutic response to PPI in NERD. [37].

The ability of NBI to depict small erosive foci could also increase consistency in the grading of erosive disease (GERD). On NBI, the limit between the squamous and columnar epithelium is clearly demarcated. Inflamed mucosal breaks appear dark brown, corresponding to the crowding of capillaries. This provides a sharp contrast to the greenish featureless epithelium. We find a classical appearance of minimal change esophagitis on NBI in a subset of patients with normal WLE (Fig. 6.4a–c). This includes a central fine ridge above the Z line, with plenty of dilated intrapapillary capillary loops (IPCLs) arranged in a linear fashion giving an inverted fir tree appearance, which resolves on PPI therapy [38]. In a recent comparative study of endoscopic images of 230 patients by WLE and NBI, both intra- and interobserver reproducibilities in grading esophagitis were improved with NBI (kappa 0.62 vs. 0.45) [39].

It appears reasonable to infer that a subset of patients with NERD would have minimal change esophagitis, which would respond therefore to PPI therapy. NBI endoscopy would thereby substantially improve our ability to predict therapeutic response in patients with reflux disease and optimize therapy.

There are still some limitations on the routine use of these endoscopic criteria in clinical practice. The assessment of dilated and tortuous IPCLs could be subjective, and objective manual counting of IPCLs is time consuming and complicated, as only a small area can be seen at one time.

Feasibility of FICE/I-Scan for the Diagnosis of GERD

These post-processing systems have been recently evaluated for the detection of mucosal breaks in GERD. Publications are limited.

In a study of 50 patients with reflux symptoms, the detection rates of mucosal rates improved with i-scan. The degree of esophagitis could be upgraded in 10% of cases [40]. A similar small study with FICE has shown higher sensitivity, NPV, and accuracy than WLE. However, the interobserver agreement was poor [41].

NBI Endoscopy in Barrett's Esophagus

Barrett's esophagus (BE) is a known premalignant lesion and has been attributed to the increasing incidence of esophageal adenocarcinoma, especially in the western world. Accordingly, regular surveillance of BE with random four-quadrant biopsies every 1–2 cm has been the standard practice. However, the distribution of dysplasia within BE is patchy and not clearly visible with WLE. The random biopsy technique is thus suboptimal and subject to sampling error.

The role of NBI in detection of BE and early cancer has been evaluated in quite a number of studies. A spectrum of changes from columnar epithelium (CLE) to high-grade dysplasia (HGD) and malignancy has been described.

Kara et al. classified Barrett's according to the mucosal pattern (flat, villous/gyrus, irregular), vascular pattern (regular, irregular, long branched), and the presence of abnormal blood vessels. Intestinal metaplasia was associated with the villous/gyrus patterns in 80% of cases and a flat mucosa in 20% of cases. On the other hand, high-grade dysplasia was characterized by irregular/disrupted mucosal and vascular patterns with abnormal blood vessels [42].

Sharma et al. used a simplified version with mucosal (ridged/villous, regular, irregular) and vascular (normal and abnormal) patterns. Here the ridged/villous pattern had a sensitivity, specificity, and PPV of 93.5%, 85%, and 94.7%, respectively, for the diagnosis of SIM. The distorted vascular pattern had a sensitivity and specificity of 100% and 98.7% [43].

Goda et al. used a more elaborate classification of the mucosal patterns into round/oval, long, straight, villous, cerebriform, and irregular and vasculature into honeycomb, vine-like, coiled, ivy-like, and irregular [44].

Singh et al. have recently proposed a combined classification based on both the mucosal and vascular patterns: (1) Pattern A, round pits and regular vasculature; (2) Pattern B, villous/ridged pits and regular vasculature; (3) Pattern C, absent pits but regular microvasculature; and (4) Pattern D, distorted pits with irregular microvasculature. Pattern A had a high PPV (100%) and NPV (97%) for CLE without SIM. Patterns B and C were indicative of SIM. Pattern D had a PPV and NPV of 81% and 99%, respectively, for high-grade dysplasia [45].

A recent meta-analysis assessed the accuracy of NBI for the characterization of dysplasia in BE with histopathology, in which 446 patients with 2194 lesions were assessed. It revealed a high diagnostic precision for HGD with a pooled sensitivity, specificity, diagnostic accuracy, and AUC revealed of 0.95 (95%CI 0.87–1.0), 0.65 (95% CI 0.52–0.78), 37.53 (95% CI 6.50–217.62), and 0.88 (SE 0.08), respectively. NBI was also able to characterize SIM with high sensitivity, but the specificity was poor [46].

Although these studies have shown promising results for NBI in detection of intestinal metaplasia and HGD, all were performed by experts in single centers and/or involved relatively small numbers of patients. By contrast, a study comparing NBI, indigo carmine chromoendoscopy, and acetic acid chromoendoscopy found no benefit from the enhanced imaging methods in identifying early neoplasia in Barrett's esophagus [47].

NBI vs. WLE in BE

Head-to-head comparison of NBI and conventional WLE in BE has been done in terms of sensitivity, specificity, diagnostic accuracy, and image quality.

Hamamoto et al. reported improved visualization of important structures with NBI. They used a scoring system of 0–4 to grade the quality of images. The squamocolumnar junction was visualized with a score of >3 in 57% of NBI compared to 17% with WLE ($p = 0.0002$). The blood vessel and CLE observation was also higher with NBI (100% vs. 80%) [48]. Curvers et al. also reported significantly better image quality with NBI compared to WLE (11.3 vs. 10.9 on visual analog scale; $p = 0.01$). Interestingly however, the diagnostic yield of neoplasia did not improve (81% vs. 83%) [49]. Singh et al. in a recent study found a significant difference between NBI and WLE in the detection of high-grade dysplasia (95% vs. 62.5% $p < 0.006$). In this study, a combination of WLE with NBI and magnification achieved a sensitivity, specificity, and accuracy of 90.2, 95, and 91.7% [50].

We find that a majority of studies comparing NBI with WLE and other modalities appear favorable for NBI. However, some interobserver studies have questioned the additional value of NBI for detection of high-grade dysplasia. NBI does appear to be operator experience dependent, and a recent study found NBI to be of limited value in BE with endoscopists in general practice [51].

In conclusion, the primary advantage of NBI is the detection of advanced dysplasia using fewer biopsy samples compared to surveillance WLE and four-quadrant biopsy. Wolfsen et al. reported 57% detection of dysplasia compared with 43% with conventional WLE and random biopsies. Additionally, the number of biopsy specimens in the four-quadrant group was much higher than targeted with NBI (mean 8.5 vs. 4.7) [52].

Autofluorescence Imaging

Autofluorescence imaging (AFI) is based on the detection of the relative concentration of endogenous fluorophores and fluorescence emission between healthy and neoplastic tissue. The use of AFI in GERD is primarily as a wide area functional imaging of Barrett's mucosa for identification of dysplastic areas [53].

Two in vivo autofluorescence-based endoscopic techniques have been investigated for detecting early neoplasia in BE:

1. Light-induced fluorescence spectroscopy (LIFS)

Autofluorescence Endoscopy

LIFS

LIFS can accurately distinguish BE with high-grade intraepithelial neoplasia (HGIN) from nondysplastic BE. An important drawback is that it only samples a small area of mucosa, making it impractical as a surveillance tool [54].

A few studies have shown improved detection of high-grade dysplasia and detection of additional cases on AFL compared to WLE with four-quadrant biopsies. The sensitivity and PPV, however, are poor, with unacceptably high false positives [55].

However, studies suggest that by combining AFI with another imaging technique (e.g., narrow-band imaging), false-positive rate can be reduced to 10–26% [56, 57].

As such, the role of AFI as a stand-alone technique for BE appears remote.

Endoscopic Trimodal Imaging (ETMI)

The ETMI system (XGIF-Q240/GIF-FQ260FZ; Olympus, Tokyo) incorporates high-resolution WLE together with AFI and NBI modalities which can be used in tandem. The improved sensitivity and specificity of the combined technique are primarily attributable to reduction of the false positivity of AFI [53].

This has been the primary intention of the studies of trimodal imaging in BE. Kara et al. first reported a significant reduction of false-positive AFI with trimodal imaging [56]. In a similar multicenter trial, Curvers et al. found that AFI could identify all cases with HGD, and false positivity was reduced by NBI from 81 to 26% [58]. The same group has recently reported improved detection of early neoplasia with ETMI compared to WLE. Here again, NBI reduced the false positivity of AFI but did misclassify 17% of cases [59].

Very interestingly, the results were not repeated when the procedures were performed by general endoscopists in the community setting, and the detection of dysplasia did not improve with ETMI [57].

Optical Biopsy (Confocal Endomicroscopy)

Confocal endomicroscopy (CLE) and endocytoscopy allow subsurface analysis of the gastrointestinal mucosa using the principle of optical sectioning. This enables real-time in vivo histology during ongoing endoscopy. Endomicroscopy and endocytoscopy dramatically expand the imaging capabilities of flexible endoscopy by their ability to obtain "optical biopsies" of nearly any accessible endoluminal surface. The current CLE incorporates a confocal laser microscope into the tip of a flexible endoscope (Pentax EC 3830FK, Tokyo, Japan). A probe-based confocal endomicroscope (Cellvizio, Mauna Kea Technologies, France) is also available.

There is limited full-length publications on the use of CLE in BE, but numerous abstracts are being presented at the GI conferences [60].

The main difference between CLE and endocytoscopy is that endocytoscopy is based solely on high-level magnification using optical lenses. Therefore, because there is no confocal plane, only the very superficial layer of the mucosa can be imaged. In addition, the lens must come into direct contact with the tissue being examined [61].

Becker et al. reported significantly higher microvessel density in neoplastic BE compared to nonneoplastic (23.6% vs. 14.2%; $p > 0.001$) on CLE [62].

Kiesslich and colleagues in a study of 63 patients with BE demonstrated good correlation between in vivo histology and conventional histology in normal squamous vis-a-vis gastric and Barrett's epithelium. A confocal classification system to predict the histopathology of the distal esophagus was also proposed.

Nondysplastic BE was characterized by regular villous-like epithelium with dark goblet cells. An increase in the number of dark cells with an irregular border was consistent with BE-associated neoplasia. The loss of regular basement membrane integrity and disruption of the villous epithelial structure suggested HGD/CA [63].

As with new technologies, CLE will need time to move from the research arena into routine clinical practice [64]. However, initial results for the prediction of dysplasia in Barrett's real time are promising [65].

Newer Imaging Advancements [66, 67]

Spectroscopic techniques such as light-scattering spectroscopy and Raman spectroscopy carry diagnostic information on the microstructural and molecular composition of tissues, which enables early detection of dysplasia. Similarly, peptides have been used as molecular probes that can be fluorescence tagged and can identify cell surface targets/molecular markers of neoplasia in BE. The results are promising. These technological advances have helped circumvent the limitation of WLE in reflux disease by (a) improved detection of subtle irregularities, (b) characterization of anomalies, and (c) possible optical biopsies providing real-time diagnosis [68]. However, these novel technologies are very much in the experimental stage and beyond the scope of this review.

Endoscopic Therapies for GERD

The endoluminal treatment of GERD is evolving and may have the potential to decrease the need for long-term antisecretory medications in selected patients.

The aim of endoscopic treatment is to create an antireflux barrier and reduce esophageal exposure to refluxate. This can be achieved by:

1. Improving the gastroesophageal flap valve that serves as a mechanical barrier to reflux
2. Reducing lower esophageal sphincter relaxation
3. Remodeling the smooth muscle at the gastroesophageal junction
4. Increasing lower esophageal sphincter length [69]

Indication for Endoscopic Therapy

Patients who may be candidates for endoscopic GERD therapy include:

1. Patients with refractory GERD, which is defined as persistent heartburn despite escalating doses of proton pump inhibitors, or residual regurgitation without heartburn symptoms while on PPIs. Esophageal pH monitoring while on PPIs to confirm increased esophageal acid exposure is mandatory in such patients.
2. Patients with bile acid reflux or non-acid reflux that has been confirmed by impedance testing.
3. Patients who are intolerant of PPIs or wish to stop drug therapy due to concerns about long-term side effects.
4. Patients who are concerned about potential side effects of antireflux surgery, such as dysphagia or gas/bloat.
5. Patients with symptomatic documented GERD following fundoplication.

In contrast, the following groups of patients are not candidates for any from endoscopic therapy for GERD:

- Patients who do not respond to PPI therapy, who have negative esophageal pH studies, and whose symptoms do not temporally correlate with acid events seen on pH monitoring probably do not have GERD and should **not** be offered endoscopic or surgical therapy for GERD.
- Patients with large, fixed hiatal hernias and esophageal foreshortening are not good candidates for endoscopic therapy, due to a high risk of technical failure.

Endoscopic Devices for Treatment of GERD

Various types of devices have been developed for the endoscopic treatment of gastroesophageal reflux disease (GERD), using approaches such as sewing, transmural fasteners, endoscopic staplers, and thermal treatment (Table 6.2).

EndoCinch The Bard EndoCinch was the first endoscopic sewing device approved by the US Food and Drug Administration (FDA) in April 2000. It has the best safety profile among the endoscopic sewing and full-thickness plication devices. Prospective observational studies in adults and children have shown mixed results, with symptomatic success rates ranging from 20 to 82% after at least 1 year of follow-up [70–73].

Adverse events noted in studies of EndoCinch included pharyngitis, vomiting, abdominal pain, mucosal tears, microperforation, bleeding, dysphagia, bronchospasm, and adverse reactions to sedation [74].

EsophyX The EndoGastric Solutions EsophyX EndoLuminal Fundoplication System is based on the principle to restore angle of His at the gastroesophageal

Table 6.2 Endoscopic devices for treatment of GERD

Devices that are currently commercially available	EndoCinch
	EsophyX
	Stretta procedure (radiofrequency treatment for GERD)
Devices that are being studied for the treatment of GERD	SRS endoscopic stapling system
Devices that are no longer or never became commercially available	Endoscopic suturing device
	NDO Plicator
	Syntheon AntiReflux device
	His-wiz device
	Enteryx procedure
	Gatekeeper reflux repair system
	Durasphere GR

junction. It affixes tissue from the GEJ to the fundus to create a neogastroesophageal valve. Efficacy of EsophyX was tested in the largest multicenter prospective study with a one-year follow-up and included 86 patients, 84 of whom successfully underwent the procedure. Objective parameters that were examined included esophageal acid exposure, which improved in 61% of patients, and mean lower esophageal sphincter pressure, which increased significantly from 12 mmHg pre-procedure to 18 mmHg post-procedure [75].

Radio Frequency Energy (Stretta Procedure) In this procedure radio frequency (RF) energy is delivered via endoscopic needles placed in the tissues surrounding the lower esophageal sphincter with constant tissue temperature monitoring to a prefixed target temperature. The putative mechanisms for efficacy include increased thickness of the LES muscle, decreased distensibility of the LES without fibrosis, and decreased frequency of TLESRs.

Many studies have demonstrated efficacy of radio frequency treatment for gastroesophageal reflux disease. Overall, 50–80% of patients have reported satisfactory symptom control or cessation of proton pump inhibitor (PPI) therapy in studies with average follow-up periods of 1–3 years [76–79].

An Italian study reported 48 months follow-up data for 56 out of 69 patients undergoing Stretta procedure. RF treatment significantly improved heartburn scores, GERD-specific quality-of-life scores, and general quality-of-life scores at 24 and 48 months in 52 out of 56 patients (92.8%); 72.3% were completely off PPIs [80].

We have recently demonstrated that the application of electrical stimulation therapy (EST) using a pacemaker significantly and consistently increases the lower esophageal sphincter (LES) pressure [81]. However, no endoscopic therapy has been completely effective in normalizing acid exposure, healing esophagitis, controlling reflux symptoms, or allowing patients to be off of all of their antisecretory medications.

Studies evaluating various endoscopic techniques for the treatment of GERD have significant limitations. More data from prospective, randomized, sham-controlled studies with adequate numbers of subjects is required. Effect of the various endoluminal treatments on esophageal tissue and the durability of response are major factors that are areas for further improvement and are important in achieving better clinical outcomes. If endoscopic treatments are to prove beneficial for patients with GERD, then devices and techniques need to be optimized and evaluated in well-designed clinical trials.

Thus, the endoscope definitely is a tool to not only diagnose and assess the patient with GERD but could also become the mode of therapy for the future. Needless to say, well-designed, independent comparative clinical trials with long-term follow-up are required before endoluminal therapy comes to clinical practice.

Conclusion

High-definition, high-resolution endoscopy enables direct visualization of the esophageal and gastric mucosa and allows tissue sampling for histology. GERD is the most common indication for endoscopy. Improved detection of GERD and surveillance of BE have now become essential in the background of rising incidence worldwide.

Standard white light endoscopy does have some limitations. Novel-enhanced imaging technology attempts to circumvent these limitations, and the results appear promising. NBI has been evaluated extensively and appears to be a useful adjunct to WLE for identification of minimal change esophagitis and for the targeted investigation of suspicious areas in BE. There is considerable evidence that NBI would help target endoscopic biopsies and delineate resection margins during endotherapy of dysplastic areas. We would recommend routine usage for detection of high-grade dysplasia in Barrett's esophagus. The days of random four-quadrant biopsies may well be over.

The primary limitation as with all new technologies is the lack of sufficiently validated and standardized classification systems and the limited number of randomized controlled trials. Additionally, most of these are conducted at tertiary care specialized centers. Routine clinical practice and cost-effectiveness remain to be tested or achieved.

References

1. Dent J, El-Serag HB, Wallander MA, Johansson S. Epidemiology of gastro–oesophageal reflux disease: a systematic review. Gut. 2005;54:710–7.
2. Fock KM, Talley NJ, Fass R, Goh KL, Katelaris P, Hunt R, et al. Asia-Pacific consensus on the management of gastroesophageal reflux disease: update. J Gastroenterol Hepatol. 2008;23(1):8–22.
3. Bruley Des Varannes S, Marek L, Humeau B, Lecasble M, Colin R. Gastroesophageal reflux disease in primary care: prevalence, epidemiology and quality of life of patients. Gastroenterol Clin Biol. 2006;30:364–70.

4. Wahlqvist P, Karlsson M, Johnson D, Carlsson J, Bolge SC, Wallander MA. Relationship between symptom load of gastro-oesophageal reflux disease and health-related quality of life, work productivity, resource utilization and concomitant diseases: survey of a US cohort. Aliment Pharmacol Ther. 2008;27(10):960–70.
5. An evidence-based appraisal of reflux disease management: the Genval workshop report [no authors listed]. Gut. 1999; 44 (Suppl 2):S1–16.
6. Kahrilas PJ, Shaheen NJ, Vaezi M. AGAI medical position panel on GERD management. AGAI medical position statement: management of gastroesophageal reflux disease. Gastroenterology. 2008;135:1383–91.
7. Fitzgerald RC, di Pietro M, Ragunath K, Ang Y, Kang JY, Watson P, et al. British Society of Gastroenterology guidelines on the diagnosis and management of Barrett's oesophagus. Gut. 2014;63:7–42.
8. Richter JE. Severe reflux esophagitis. Gastrointest Endosc Clin North Am. 1994;4:677–98.
9. Nayer DW, Vaezi MF. Classification of esophagitis: who needs it? Gastrointest Endosc. 2004;60:253.
10. Lundell LR, Dent J, Bennett JR, et al. Endoscopic assessment of oesophagitis: clinical and functional correlates and further validation of the Los Angeles classification. Gut. 1999;45:172–80.
11. Falk GW, Fennerty BF, Rothstein RI. AGA institute technical review on the use of endoscopic therapy for gastroesophageal reflux disease. Gastroenterology. 2006;131:1315–36.
12. Wani S, Sharma P. Changing the "contrast" in GERD. Gastrointest Endosc. 2007;66(2):237–9.
13. Nakamura T, Shirakawa K, Masuyama H, Sugaya H, Terano A. Minimal change oesophagitis: a disease with characteristic differences to erosive esophagitis. Aliment Pharmacol Ther. 2005;21(Suppl 2):19–26.
14. Spechler SJ. Clinical practice. Barrett's esophagus N Engl J Med. 2002;346:836–42.
15. Falk GW, Rice TW, Goldblum JR, Richter JE. Jumbo biopsy forceps protocol still misses unsuspected cancer in Barrett's esophagus with high grade dysplasia. Gastrointest Endosc. 1999;49:170–6.
16. Kim SL, Waring JP, Spechler SJ, Sampliner RE, Doos WG, Krol WF, et al. Diagnostic inconsistencies in Barrett's esophagus. Department of Veterans Affairs Gastroesophageal Reflux Study Group. Gastroenterology. 1994;107:945–9.
17. Bergman JJ, Tytgat GN. New developments in the endoscopic surveillance of Barrett's oesophagus. Gut. 2005;(Suppl I):54, 138–142.
18. Reddymasu SC, Sharma P. Advances in endoscopic imaging of the oesophagus. Gastroenterol Clin N Am. 2008;37:763–74.
19. Kiesslich R, Kanzler S, Vieth M, Moehler M, Neidig J, Thanka Nadar BJ, et al. Minimal change esophagitis: prospective comparison of endoscopic and histological markers between patients with non-erosive reflux disease and normal controls using magnifying endoscopy. Dig Dis. 2004;22:221–7.
20. Banerjee R, Reddy DN. Minimal-change esophagitis on narrow-band imaging. Clin Gastroenterol Hepatol. 2008;6(8):A26.
21. Guelrud M, Herrera I, Essenfeld H, Castro J. Enhanced magnification endoscopy: a new technique to identify specialized intestinal metaplasia in Barrett's esophagus. Gastrointest Endosc. 2001;53:559–65.
22. Endo T, Awakawa T, Takahashi H, Arimura Y, Itoh F, Yamashita K, et al. Classification of Barrett's epithelium by magnifying endoscopy. Gastrointest Endosc. 2002;55:641–7.
23. Sharma P, Weston AP, Topalovski M, Cherian R, Bhattacharyya A, Sampliner RE. Magnification chromoendoscopy for the detection of intestinal metaplasia and dysplasia in Barrett's oesophagus. Gut. 2003;52:24–7.
24. Yoshikawa I, Yamasaki M, Yamasaki T, Kume K, Otsuki M. Lugol chromoendoscopy as a diagnostic tool in so−called endoscopy−negative GERD. Gastrointest Endosc. 2005;62:698–703.
25. Canto MI, Setrakian S, Willis J, Chak A, Petras R, Powe NR, et al. Methylene blue-directed biopsies improve detection of intestinal metaplasia and dysplasia in Barrett's esophagus. Gastrointest Endosc. 2000;51:560–8.

26. Horwhat JD, Maydonovitch CL, Ramos F, Colina R, Gaertner E, Lee H, et al. A randomized comparison of methylene blue-directed biopsy versus conventional four-quadrant biopsy for the detection of intestinal metaplasia and dysplasia in patients with long-segment Barrett's esophagus. Am J Gastroenterol. 2008;103:546–54.
27. Olliver JR, Wild CP, Sahay P, Dexter S, Hardie LJ. Chromoendoscopy with methylene blue and associated DNA damage in Barrett's oesophagus. Lancet. 2003;362:373–4.
28. Curvers W, Baak L, Kiesslich R, Van Oijen A, Rabenstein T, Ragunath K, et al. Chromoendoscopy and narrow-band imaging compared with high-resolution magnification endoscopy in Barrett's esophagus. Gastroenterology. 2008;134:670–9.
29. Kara MA, Peters FP, Rosmolen WD, Krishnadath KK, ten Kate FJ, Fockens P, et al. High-resolution endoscopy plus chromoendoscopy or narrow-band imaging in Barrett's esophagus: a prospective randomized crossover study. Endoscopy. 2005;37:929–36.
30. Banerjee R, Reddy DN. Advanced gastrointestinal endoscopy: a primer on narrow band imaging. Hyderabad: Paras Medical Publisher; 2009. p. 5–26.
31. Kumagai Y, Inoue H, Nagai K, Kawano T, Iwai T. Magnifying endoscopy, stereoscopic microscopy, and the microvascular architecture of superficial esophageal carcinoma. Endoscopy. 2002;34:369–75.
32. Yoshida T, Inoue H, Usui S, Satodate H, Fukami N, Kudo SE. Narrow-band imaging system with magnifying endoscopy for superficial esophageal lesions. Gastrointest Endosc. 2004 Feb;59(2):288–95.
33. Dent J, Armstrong D, Delaney B, Moayyedi P, Talley NJ, Vakil N. Symptom evaluation in reflux disease: workshop background, processes, terminology, recommendations and discussion outputs. Gut. 2004;53(Suppl 4):1–24.
34. Sharma P, Wani S, Bansal A, Hall S, Puli S, Mathur S, et al. A feasibility trial of narrow band imaging endoscopy in patients with gasdtroesophageal reflux disease. Gastroenterology. 2007;133:454–64.
35. Banerjee PN, Ramchandani M, Tandan M, Guduru V. Narrow band imaging (NBI) can detect minimal changes in non erosive reflux disease (NERD) which resolve with PPI therapy. Gastrointest Endosc. 69(5):AB356.
36. Fock KM, Teo EK, Ang T, Tan JY, Law NM. The utility of narrow band imaging in improving the endoscopic diagnosis of gastroesophageal disease. Clin Gastroenterol Hepatol. 2009;7(1):54–9.
37. Tseng PH, Chen CC, Chiu HM, Liao WC, Wu MS, Lin JT, et al. Performance of narrow band imaging and magnification endoscopy in the prediction of therapeutic response in patients with gastroesophageal reflux disease. J Clin Gastroenterol. 2010.; [Epub ahead of print]
38. Lee YC, Lin JT, Chiu HM, Liao WC, Chen CC, Tu CH, et al. Intraobserver and interobserver consistency for grading esophagitis with narrow-band imaging. Gastrointest Endosc. 2007;66(2):230–6.
39. Banerjee R, Reddy DN. Minimal-change esophagitis on narrow band imaging. Clin Gastroenterol Hepatol. 2008;6(8):A26.
40. Hoffman A, Basting N, Goetz M, Tresch A, Mudter J, Biesterfeld S, et al. High definition endoscopy with i-scan and Lugol's solution for more precise detection of mucosal breaks in patients with reflux symptoms. Endoscopy. 2009;41:107–12.
41. Chaiteerakij R, Geratikornsupuk N, Tangmankongworakoon N, et al. Efficacy of intelligent chromo endoscopy for detection of minimal mucosal breaks in patients with typical reflux symptoms of gastroesophageal reflux disease. Gastrointest Endosc. 2008;67:AB86.
42. Kara MA, Ennahachi M, Fockens P, ten Kate FJ, Bergman JJ. Detection and classification of the mucosal and vascular patterns (mucosal morphology) in Barrett's esophagus by using narrow band imaging. Gastrointest Endosc. 2006;64(2):155–66.
43. Sharma P, Bansal A, Mathur S, Wani S, Cherian R, McGregor D, et al. The utility of a novel narrow band imaging endoscopy system in patients with Barrett's esophagus. Gastrointest Endosc. 2006;64(2):167–75.
44. Goda K, Tajiri H, Ikegami M, Urashima M, Nakayoshi T, Kaise M. Usefulness of magnifying endoscopy with narrow band imaging for the detection of specialized intestinal

metaplasia in columnar-lined esophagus and Barrett's adenocarcinoma. Gastrointest Endosc. 2007;65(1):36–46.

45. Singh R, Anagnostopoulos GK, Yao K, Karageorgiou H, Fortun PJ, Shonde A, et al. Narrow-band imaging with magnification in Barrett's esophagus: validation of a simplified grading system of mucosal morphology patterns against histology. Endoscopy. 2008;40(6):457–63.

46. Mannath J, Subramanian V, Hawkey CJ, Ragunath K. Narrow band imaging for characterization of HGD and SIM in Barrett's esophagus: a meta-analysis. Endoscopy. 2010;42:351–9.

47. Curvers W, Baak L, Kiesslich R, Van Oijen A, Rabenstein T, Ragunath K, et al. Chromoendoscopy and narrow-band imaging compared with high-resolution magnification endoscopy in Barrett's esophagus. Gastroenterology. 2008;134:670–9.

48. Hamamoto Y, Endo T, Nosho K, Arimura Y, Sato M, Imai K. Usefulness of narrow-band imaging endoscopy for diagnosis of Barrett's esophagus. J Gastroenterol. 2004;39(1):14–20.

49. Curvers WL, Bohmer CJ, Mallant-Hent RC, Naber AH, Ponsioen CI, Ragunath K, et al. Mucosal morphology in Barrett's esophagus: interobserver agreement and role of narrow band imaging. Endoscopy. 2008;40(10):799–805.

50. Singh R, Karageorgiou H, Owen V, Garsed K, Fortun PJ, Fogden E, et al. Comparison of high-resolution magnification narrow-band imaging and white-light endoscopy in the prediction of histology in Barrett's oesophagus. Scand J Gastroenterol. 2009;44(1):85–92.

51. Silva FB, Dinis-Ribeiro M, Vieth M, Rabenstein T, Goda K, Kiesslich R, et al. Endoscopic assessment and grading of Barrett's esophagus using magnification endoscopy and narrow-band imaging: accuracy and interobserver agreement of different classification systems (with videos). Gastrointest Endosc. 2011;73(1):7–14.

52. Wolfsen HC, Crook JE, Krishna M, Achem SR, Devault KR, Bouras EP, et al. Prospective, controlled tandem endoscopy study of narrow band imaging for dysplasia detection in Barrett's Esophagus. Gastroenterology. 2008 Jul;135(1):24–31.

53. Falk GW. Autofluorescence endoscopy. Gastrointest Endosc Clin N Am. 2009 Apr;19(2):209–20.

54. Georgakoudi I, Jacobson BC, Van Dam J, Backman V, Wallace MB, Müller MG, et al. Fluorescence, reflectance, and light-scattering spectroscopy for evaluating dysplasia in patients with Barrett's esophagus. Gastroenterology. 2001;120(7):1620–9.

55. Kara MA, Peters FP, Ten Kate FJ, Van Deventer SJ, Fockens P, Bergman JJ. Endoscopic video autofluorescence imaging may improve the detection of early neoplasia in patients with Barrett's esophagus. Gastrointest Endosc. 2005;61(6):679–85.

56. Kara MA, Peters FP, Fockens P, Kate FJ, Bergman JJ. Endoscopic video-autofluorescence imaging followed by narrow band imaging for detecting early neoplasia in Barrett's esophagus. Gastrointest Endosc. 2006;64(2):176–85.

57. Curvers WL, Van Vilsteren FG, Baak LC, Böhmer C, Mallant-Hent RC, Naber AH, et al. Endoscopic trimodal imaging versus standard video endoscopy for detection of early Barrett's neoplasia: a multicenter, randomized, crossover study in general practice. Gastrointest Endosc. 2011;73(2):195–203.

58. Curvers WL, Singh R, Song LM, Wolfsen HC, Ragunath K, Wang K, et al. Endoscopic tri-modal imaging for detection of early neoplasia in Barrett's oesophagus: a multi-centre feasibility study using high-resolution endoscopy, autofluorescence imaging and narrow band imaging incorporated in one endoscopy system. Gut. 2008;57(2):167–72.

59. Curvers WL, Herrero LA, Wallace MB, Wong Kee Song LM, Ragunath K, Wolfsen HC, et al. Endoscopic tri-modal imaging is more effective than standard endoscopy in identifying early-stage neoplasia in Barrett's esophagus. Gastroenterology. 2010;139(4):1106–14.

60. Nguyen NQ, Leong RW. Current application of confocal endomicroscopy in gastrointestinal disorders. J Gastroenterol Hepatol. 2008;23(10):1483–91.

61. Tomizawa Y, Iyer PG, Wongkeesong LM, Buttar NS, Lutzke LS, Wu TT, Wang KK. Assessment of the diagnostic performance and interobserver variability of endocytoscopy in Barrett's esophagus: a pilot ex-vivo study. World J Gastroenterol. 2013;19(46):8652–8.

62. Becker V, Vieth M, Bajbouj M, Schmid RM, Meining A. Confocal laser scanning fluorescence microscopy for in vivo determination of microvessel density in Barrett's esophagus. Endoscopy. 2008;40(11):888–91.
63. Kiesslich R, Gossner L, Goetz M, Dahlmann A, Vieth M, Stolte M, et al. In vivo histology of Barrett's esophagus and associated neoplasia by confocal laser endomicroscopy. Clin Gastroenterol Hepatol. 2006;4(8):979–87.
64. Bajbouj M, Vieth M, Rösch T, Miehlke S, Becker V, Anders M, et al. Probe-based confocal laser endomicroscopy compared with standard four-quadrant biopsy for evaluation of neoplasia in Barrett's esophagus. Endoscopy. 2010;42(6):435–40.
65. Canto MI. Endomicroscopy of Barrett's Esophagus. Gastroenterol Clin N Am. 2010;39(4):759–69.
66. Wallace MB, Wax A, Roberts DN, Graf RN. Reflectance spectroscopy. Gastrointest Endosc Clin N Am. 2009 Apr;19(2):233–42.
67. Li M, Anastassiades CP, Joshi B, Komarck CM, Piraka C, Elmunzer BJ, et al. Affinity peptide for targeted detection of dysplasia in Barrett's esophagus. Gastroenterology. 2010;139(5):1472–80.
68. Banerjee R, Reddy DN. Enhanced endoscopic imaging and gastroesophageal reflux disease. Indian J Gastroenterol. 2011;30(5):193–200.
69. Jafri SM, Arora G, Triadafilopoulos G. What is left of the endoscopic antireflux devices? Curr Opin Gastroenterol. 2009;25(4):352–7.
70. Schiefke I, Zabel-Langhennig A, Neumann S, Feisthammel J, Moessner J, Caca K. Long term failure of endoscopic gastroplication (EndoCinch). Gut. 2005;54(6):752–8.
71. Chen YK, Raijman I, Ben-Menachem T, Starpoli AA, Liu J, Pazwash H, et al. Long-term outcomes of endoluminal gastroplication: a U.S. multicenter trial. Gastrointest Endosc. 2005;61(6):659–67.
72. Arts J, Lerut T, Rutgeerts P, Sifrim D, Janssens J, Tack J. A one-year follow-up study of endoluminal gastroplication (Endocinch) in GERD patients refractory to proton pump inhibitor therapy. Dig Dis Sci. 2005;50(2):351–6.
73. Schwartz MP, Wellink H, Gooszen HG, Conchillo JM, Samsom M, Smout AJ. Endoscopic gastroplication for the treatment of gastro-oesophageal reflux disease: a randomised, sham-controlled trial. Gut. 2007;56(1):20–8.
74. Montgomery M, Håkanson B, Ljungqvist O, Ahlman B, Thorell A. Twelve months' follow-up after treatment with the EndoCinch endoscopic technique for gastro-oesophageal reflux disease: a randomized, placebo-controlled study. Scand J Gastroenterol. 2006;41(12):1382–9.
75. Cadière GB, Buset M, Muls V, Rajan A, Rösch T, Eckardt AJ, et al. Antireflux transoral incisionless fundoplication using EsophyX: 12-month results of a prospective multicenter study. World J Surg. 2008;32(8):1676–88.
76. Wolfsen HC, Richards WO. The Stretta procedure for the treatment of GERD: a registry of 558 patients. J Laparoendosc Adv Surg Tech A. 2002;12(6):395–402.
77. Torquati A, Houston HL, Kaiser J, Holzman MD, Richards WO. Long-term follow-up study of the Stretta procedure for the treatment of gastroesophageal reflux disease. Surg Endosc. 2004;18(10):1475–9.
78. White B, Jeansonne LO, Cook M, Chavarriaga LF, Goldenberg EA, Davis SS, et al. Use of endoluminal antireflux therapies for obese patients with GERD. Obes Surg. 2009;19(6):783–7.
79. Corley DA, Katz P, Wo JM, Stefan A, Patti M, Rothstein R, et al. Improvement of gastroesophageal reflux symptoms after radiofrequency energy: a randomized, sham-controlled trial. Gastroenterology. 2003;125(3):668–76.
80. Dughera L, Navino M, Cassolino P, De Cento M, Cacciotella L, Cisarò F, et al. Long-term results of radiofrequency energy delivery for the treatment of GERD: results of a prospective 48-month study. Diagn Ther Endosc. 2011;2011:507157.
81. Banerjee R, Pratap N, Kalpala R, Reddy DN. Effect of electrical stimulation of the lower esophageal sphincter using endoscopically implanted temporary stimulation leads in patients with reflux disease. Surg Endosc. 2014 Mar;28(3):1003–9.

Michio Hongo and Julius Carlo R. Rustia

Abstract

Evidence shows that gastroesophageal reflux disease (GERD) is rapidly rising in Asia. Recent globalization of economies and the associated lifestyle changes may have tipped the balance in favor of the development of GERD. Medical treatment consisting of lifestyle and dietary modifications and pharmacologic therapy are the mainstays of treatment. Only elevation of the head of the bed, left lateral decubitus positioning, and weight loss have been associated with GERD improvement. There is insufficient evidence to support restriction of alcohol, tobacco, caffeine, spicy foods, chocolate, citrus, and carbonated drinks. Avoidance of these may help with GERD symptoms. Acid suppression therapy with PPI is still the cornerstone of pharmacologic treatment of erosive esophagitis, NERD, and extraesophageal symptoms of GERD. Adjunctive treatment with H2 antagonists, antacids, alginates, and prokinetics may be used in GERD patients refractory to PPI.

Keywords

GERD • Erosive esophagitis • Reflux esophagitis • NERD • PPI • H2RA • Prokinetics • Antacid • Alginate

M. Hongo (⊠)
Kurokawa General Hospital, Tohoku University, 60 Nishi-Hinoki, Yoshioka, Kurokawa, Miyagi 981-3682, Japan
e-mail: m-hongo@med.tohoku.ac.jp

J.C.R. Rustia
Gastroenterologist and Specialized Advanced Therapeutic Endoscopist,
Aquinas University Hospital Foundation Inc, Legazpi City, Albay, Philippines

© Springer India 2018
P. Sharma et al. (eds.), *The Rise of Acid Reflux in Asia*,
DOI 10.1007/978-81-322-0846-4_7

Introduction

Medical treatment is the mainstay of treatment of GERD and includes lifestyle and dietary modifications and pharmacologic therapy. Acid suppression therapy is the cornerstone of pharmacological treatment of GERD since the advent of H2 antagonists. Currently, proton pump inhibitors (PPIs) offer the most effective acid suppression and are used widely throughout the world for the treatment of GERD.

Lifestyle and Dietary Modification

Lifestyle interventions are part of therapy for GERD. Counseling is provided regarding weight loss, head of bed elevation, tobacco and alcohol cessation, avoidance of late-night meals, and cessation of foods that can potentially aggravate reflux. Physiologic studies show that these maneuvers enhance esophageal acid clearance, decrease acid reflux-related events, or ease heartburn symptoms [1]. However, in case-controlled studies, only elevation of the head of the bed, left lateral decubitus positioning, and weight loss have been associated with GERD improvement [1].

Studies have shown improvement in GERD symptoms and esophageal pH values with head of bed elevation using blocks or foam wedges (Table 7.1) [2–4]. Weight gain, even in subjects with a normal BMI, has been associated with new onset of GERD symptoms [5]. Morbidly obese patients have been shown to have statistically more GERD symptoms compared to nonobese subjects [6]. Weight loss has also been shown to reduce GERD symptoms [7, 8]. One large case-controlled study

Table 7.1 Efficacy of lifestyle interventions adapted from 2013 ACG guidelines for the diagnosis and management of GERD

Lifestyle intervention	Effect of intervention on GERD parameters	Sources of data	Recommendation
Weight loss	Improvement of GERD symptoms and esophageal pH	Case control	Strong recommendation for patients with BMI>25 or patients with recent weight gain
Head of bed elevation	Improved esophageal pH and symptoms	Randomized controlled trial	Head of bed elevation with foam wedge or blocks in patients with nocturnal GERD
Avoidance of late evening meals	Improved nocturnal gastric acidity but not symptoms	Case control	Avoid eating meals with high-fat content within 2–3 h of reclining
Tobacco and alcohol cessation	No change in symptoms or esophageal pH	Case control	Not recommended to improve GERD symptoms
Cessation of chocolate, caffeine, spicy foods, citrus, carbonated beverages	No studies performed	No evidence	Not routinely recommended for GERD patients. Selective elimination could be considered if patients note correlation with GERD symptoms and improvement with elimination

showed there was a 40% reduction in frequent GERD symptoms for women who reduced their BMI by 3.5 or more compared with controls [5]. Roux-en-Y gastric bypass was considered an effective method to alleviate symptoms of GERD [9].

Consumption of tobacco, chocolate, and carbonated beverages and lying in the right lateral decubitus position have been shown to decrease lower esophageal sphincter pressure (LESP), whereas consumption of alcohol, coffee, caffeine, and spicy and fatty foods had no effect. There was an increase in esophageal acid exposure times with tobacco and alcohol consumption in addition to ingestion of chocolate and fatty foods. However, tobacco and alcohol cessation were not shown to raise LESP, improve esophageal pH, or improve GERD symptoms. There have been no studies that have shown clinical improvement in GERD symptoms with cessation of coffee, caffeine, chocolate, spicy foods, citrus, carbonated beverages, fatty foods, or mint [1].

Other measures that theoretically can improve symptoms, however, have not been shown to be effective, including (1) avoidance of tight-fitting garments to prevent increasing intragastric pressure and the gastroesophageal pressure gradient, (2) promotion of salivation through oral lozenges/chewing gum to neutralize refluxed acid and increase the rate of esophageal acid clearance [10], and (3) abdominal breathing exercise to strengthen the anti-reflux barrier of the lower esophageal sphincter [11].

Pharmacologic Agents

Proton Pump Inhibitors (PPIs)

PPIs are the most potent inhibitors of gastric acid secretion by irreversibly binding to and inhibiting the H-K-ATPase pump. PPIs are most effective when taken 30 min before the first meal of the day because the amount of H-K-ATPase present in the parietal cell is greatest after a prolonged fast [12]. They are the drugs of choice as recommended by the different practice guidelines (Table 7.2).

The 2008 Asia-Pacific consensus on the management of GERD recommends 4 weeks of PPI treatment for nonerosive reflux disease (NERD) patients and 4 to 8 weeks for erosive esophagitis. PPIs at standard doses for 8 weeks relieve symptoms of GERD and heal esophagitis in up to 86% of patients with erosive esophagitis [12]. PPI therapy has been associated with superior and faster healing rates and decreased relapse rates compared with H2RAs and placebo [13].

There are no major differences in efficacy among PPIs and no consistent increase in symptom resolution or esophagitis healing rates between different dosages or dosing regimens of PPI therapy [14]. All of the PPIs, with the exception of dexlansoprazole, should be administered 30–60 min before meals to assure efficacy. Dexlansoprazole, the newest PPI available for use, is a dual delayed-release PPI licensed for use in the Asian Pacific region recently. Comparative trials of dexlansoprazole compared with lansoprazole 30 mg demonstrated superior control in

Table 7.2 Medical therapy for GERD

	Recommendations	Comments
Lifestyle changes	Weight loss, elevation of head, and left lateral decubitus position	Insufficient evidence to support restriction of alcohol, tobacco, caffeine, spicy foods, chocolate, citrus, and carbonated drinks. Avoidance of these may help with GERD symptoms
Proton pump inhibitor therapy	Drug of choice in GERD	No major differences in efficacy among PPIs
	Erosive esophagitis, 6–8 weeks at standard dose	No consistent increase in symptom resolution or esophagitis healing rates between different dosages or dosing regimens of PPI therapy
	NERD, 4 weeks at standard dose	
	Extraesophageal GERD	
	Refractory GERD	
H2 antagonists	More effective in controlling nocturnal acid secretion	Esophagitis healing rates rarely exceeded 60%
		Tachyphylaxis within 2–6 weeks
Alginates	Reduces the postprandial acid pocket in the proximal stomach	Gaviscon Double Action Liquid was found to be more effective than an antacid without alginate in controlling postprandial esophageal acid exposure
	Found to be as effective as omeprazole in the treatment of NERD	
	Decreases reflux and dyspeptic symptoms in GERD patients	
Prokinetic agents	Increases LES pressure, acid clearance, or gastric emptying	Its use as either monotherapy or adjunctive therapy to PPIs may have a role in the treatment of GERD in Asia
	Modest benefit in controlling heartburn	May cause cardiac dysrhythmias
	Unreliable efficacy in healing esophagitis	
Antacids	For episodic, primarily postprandial heartburn and intermittent (on-demand), mild GERD symptoms	Relief of heartburn within 5 min but have a short duration of effect of 30–60 min.
Other agents	Sucralfate limited only pregnant patients with GERD	Insufficient studies for *rikkunshito*, anxiolytics and antidepressants, electroacupuncture, melatonin, and anti-osteoporosis medication elcatonin
	Baclofen may be used in PPI refractory GERD patients	

esophageal pH values and better efficacy in healing esophagitis, maintenance of healing, and symptom control. There is the added convenience of being able to dose the drug any time of the day regardless of food intake [15].

Histamine 2 Receptor Antagonists (H2RAs)

H2RAs are commonly used for episodic heartburn, primarily for postprandial heartburn. However, the development of tachyphylaxis within 2–6 weeks limits their use as maintenance therapy [16].

H2RAs have a slower onset of action, reaching peak concentrations 2.5 h after dosing, but a significantly longer duration of action, lasting 4–10 h [17].

Overall esophagitis healing rates with H2RAs rarely exceeded 60% after up to 12 weeks of treatment, even when higher doses were used. Healing rates differ in individual trials depending primarily on the severity of esophagitis being treated: LA grades I and II esophagitis heal in 60–90% of patients, whereas LA grades III and IV heal in only 30–50% of patients, despite high-dose regimens [18].

The addition of bedtime H2RA has been recommended for patients with symptoms refractory to PPI. The trial use of a bedtime H2RA might be most beneficial if dosed on an as-needed basis in patients with provocable nighttime symptoms and patients with objective evidence on pH monitoring of overnight esophageal acid reflux despite optimal PPI use.

Antacids

Antacids are commonly used for episodic heartburn, primarily for postprandial heartburn [19]. They are also used for intermittent (on-demand), mild GERD symptoms that occur less than once a week [20]. Antacids neutralize gastric pH, thereby decreasing the exposure of the esophageal mucosa to gastric acid during reflux episodes. Antacids begin to provide relief of heartburn within 5 min but have a short duration of effect of 30–60 min.

Sodium Alginate

Sodium alginate is a polysaccharide derived from seaweed that forms a viscous gum that floats within the stomach and reduces the postprandial acid pocket in the proximal stomach. It was found to be as effective as omeprazole in the treatment of NERD [21]. It decreases reflux and dyspeptic symptoms in GERD patients compared with matched placebo and has a favorable benefit-risk balance [22]. An alginate-antacid combination was found to be more effective than an antacid without alginate in controlling postprandial esophageal acid exposure. Its main effectiveness relates to its co-localization with and displacement/neutralization of the postprandial acid pocket, rather than preventing mechanical reflux [23].

Prokinetics

Prokinetic drugs improve reflux symptoms by increasing LES pressure, acid clearance, or gastric emptying. However, they provide only modest benefit in controlling heartburn but have unreliable efficacy in healing esophagitis [24]. Their use as either monotherapy or adjunctive therapy to PPIs may have a role in the treatment of GERD in Asia.

Metoclopramide has been shown to increase LESP, enhance esophageal peristalsis, and augment gastric emptying [25]. It is another option in patients with incomplete response to PPI. Clinical data showing additional benefit of metoclopramide to PPI or H2RA has not been adequately studied and has not been shown to be more effective compared with combination and single therapy. In the absence of gastroparesis, there is no clear role for metoclopramide. Central nervous system side effects are drowsiness, agitation, irritability, depression, dystonic reactions, and tardive dyskinesia.

Domperidone, a peripherally acting dopamine agonist, is not approved by the US FDA but is commonly used in Asia. Monitoring for QT prolongation is performed, due to a small risk for ventricular arrhythmia and sudden cardiac death [26].

Cisapride, a serotonin (5-HT$_4$) receptor agonist, increases acetylcholine release in the myenteric plexus. It was withdrawn from the market because of serious cardiac dysrhythmias (ventricular tachycardia, ventricular fibrillation, torsades de pointes, and QT prolongation).

Itopride, a dopamine D$_2$ antagonist with antiacetylcholinesterase effect, has been recently evaluated in patients with an abnormal pH test and mild erosive reflux disease (ERD). After 30 days of treatment in an open-label study design, itopride significantly reduced the extent of esophageal acid exposure and improved GERD-related symptoms as compared to baseline values [27].

Mosapride, a newly developed 5-HT$_4$ agonist, has been shown to increase the rate of complete esophageal bolus transit and enhances esophageal bolus transit in normal controls. However, mosapride with PPI combined therapy was found not to be more effective than PPI alone as first-line therapy [28].

Bethanechol, a cholinergic agonist, is limited by flushing, blurred vision, headaches, abdominal cramps, and urinary frequency.

Baclofen

Baclofen, a GABAB agonist, is effective in GERD by its ability to reduce transient LES relaxations, thereby reducing exposure time for acid and duodenal reflux. In PPI refractory GERD patients, a trial of 5–20 mg three times a day can be considered in patients with objective documentation of continued symptomatic reflux despite optimal PPI therapy [27].

Other Treatment Options

Herbal medicines, such as *rikkunshito* [29], anxiolytics and antidepressants, electroacupuncture, melatonin, and anti-osteoporosis medication elcatonin [30], have anecdotal reports in the treatment of GERD.

Clinical Practice for GERD in ASIA: Recommendations

Non-pharmacologic therapy with lifestyle changes is easy to institute and should be advised to a patient. These include weight loss, elevation of the head of the bed, and left lateral decubitus position. There is insufficient evidence to support restriction of alcohol, tobacco, caffeine, spicy foods, chocolate, citrus, and carbonated drinks. However, avoidance of these.

Specific Pharmacologic Therapy

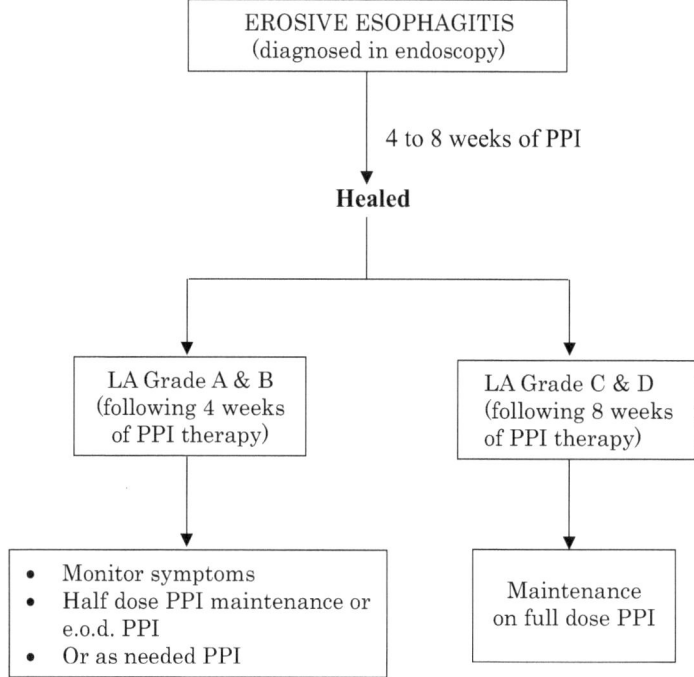

Initial Treatment

PPIs for 4–8 weeks are the most effective treatment for erosive esophagitis [19]. PPIs at standard doses for 8 weeks relieve symptoms of GERD and heal esophagitis in up to 86% of patients with erosive esophagitis [12].

Maintenance of Healing

The US FDA has approved all the PPIs, sometimes at one-half the acute dose, for maintenance therapy for mild esophagitis (LA Grade A and B). Furthermore, the 2008 Asia-Pacific consensus on the management of GERD recommends on-demand therapy defined as PPI consumption (up to once daily) when needed and for the duration desired. On-demand PPI therapy was superior to placebo in controlling GERD-related symptoms, antacids consumption, and patients' satisfaction with therapy. Patients with severe disease (daily symptoms, severe esophagitis, or complications) are put on maintenance PPI therapy indefinitely [27].

NERD

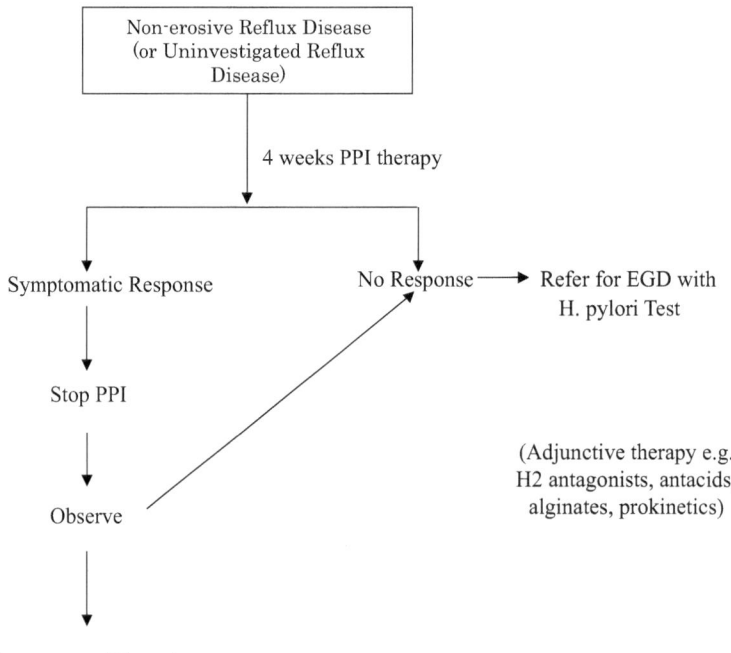

Initial Treatment

PPIs are the most effective treatment for NERD and are recommended as first-line therapy for NERD. Patients should be prescribed a minimum of 4 weeks of initial continuous therapy with a PPI [19]. PPIs demonstrate superiority in relieving heartburn symptoms in patients with NERD when compared to H2RAs [31].

Maintenance Treatment

Studies have shown that on-demand PPI therapy was superior to placebo in controlling GERD-related symptoms, antacids consumption, and patients' satisfaction with therapy [32]. Several cost-effectiveness analyses have demonstrated that on-demand treatment with a PPI is cost-effective compared with other therapeutic strategies for GERD (e.g., lifestyle therapy and antacids, H2RA therapy, step-up, step-down, as well as others) [33].

No Response to Treatment

Endoscopy should be performed at least once in patients with chronic upper gut symptoms, recognizing the imprecision of clinical diagnosis between GERD, gastric cancer, and peptic ulcer and the ability of endoscopy to provide or exclude a diagnosis and aid in tailoring therapy [19]. Based on symptoms alone, 18% of *H. pylori*-related peptic ulcers were misdiagnosed as GERD [34]. *H. pylori* testing should be considered in new patients presenting with GERD symptoms in regions with a high prevalence of gastric cancer or peptic ulcer disease [19]. H2RA for control of nocturnal acid secretion, prokinetics [27], antacids for episodic heartburn [20], and sodium alginate [21] may be also be used as adjunctive treatment in NERD patients. Clinical data showing additional benefit of prokinetics with PPI has not been adequately studied. Combination therapy of metoclopramide with H2RA has not been shown to be more effective compared with H2RA or prokinetic therapy alone [35]. Mosapride with PPI combined therapy was also found not to be more effective than PPI alone as first-line therapy [28].

Extraesophageal Treatment

The Montreal Consensus recognized established associations between GERD and asthma, chronic cough, and laryngitis while acknowledging that these disorders frequently have a multifactorial etiology and that gastroesophageal reflux may be a cofactor rather than a cause.

Patients with chronic cough and laryngitis and typical GERD symptoms should be offered twice-daily PPI therapy after exclusion of non-GERD etiologies for at least 4 months [19]. Two randomized controlled trials have shown that PPIs result in improvement of various asthma outcomes [36, 37]. However, there is insufficient evidence to recommend PPIs for routine asthma treatment when other GERD symptoms are absent [38]. The experience with treating laryngeal symptoms attributed to reflux disease is comparable. A meta-analysis of eight randomized controlled trials found that PPI therapy had no significant advantage over placebo in achieving improvement of symptoms of suspected GERD-related chronic laryngitis [39]. Park et al. demonstrated that double-dose PPI is superior to once-daily PPI in controlling chronic cough symptoms [40]. Aggressive acid suppression with twice-daily PPI for at least 4 months is warranted for the treatment of GERD-related chronic cough [41].

References

1. Kaltenbach T, Crockett S, Gerson LB. Are lifestyle measures effective in patients with gastro-esophageal reflux disease? An evidence-based approach. Arch Intern Med. 2006;166:65–71.
2. Stanciu C, Bennett JR. Effects of posture on gastro-oesophageal reflux. Digestion. 1977;15:104–9.
3. Hamilton JW, Boisen RJ, Yamamoto DT, Wagner JL, Reichelderfer M. Sleeping on a wedge diminishes exposure of the esophagus to refluxed acid. Dig Dis Sci. 1988;33(5):518–22.
4. Pollmann H, Zillessen E, Pohl J, Rosemeyer D, Abucar A, Armbrecht U, et al. Effect of elevated head position in bed in therapy of gastroesophageal reflux. Z Gastroenterol. 1996;34(Suppl 2):93–9.
5. Jacobson BC, Somers SC, Fuchs CS, Kelly CP, Camargo CA Jr. Body-mass index and symptoms of gastroesophageal reflux in women. N Engl J Med. 2006;354(22):2340–8.
6. Huseini M, Wood GC, Seiler J, Argyropoulos G, Irving BA, Gerhard GS, et al. Gastrointestinal symptoms in morbid obesity. Front Med (Lausanne). 2014;1:49.
7. Fraser-Moodie CA, Norton B, Gornall C, Magnago S, Weale AR, Holmes GK. Weight loss has an independent beneficial effect on symptoms of gastro-oesophageal reflux in patients who are overweight. Scand J Gastroenterol. 1999;34(4):337–40.
8. Mathus-Vliegen LM, Tytgat GN. Twenty-four-hour pH measurements in morbid obesity: effects of massive overweight, weight loss and gastric distension. Eur J Gastroenterol Hepatol. 1996;8:635–40.
9. El-Hadi M, Birch DW, Gill RS, Karmali S. The effect of bariatric surgery on gastroesophageal reflux disease. Can J Surg. 2014;57(2):139–44.
10. Moazzez R, Bartlett D, Anggiansah A. The effect of chewing sugar-free gum on gastro- esophageal reflux. J Dent Res. 2005 Nov;84(11):1062–5.
11. Eherer A. Management of gastroesophageal reflux disease: lifestyle modification and alternative approaches. Dig Dis. 2014;32(1–2):149–51. Epub 2014 Feb 28
12. Hunt R. Acid suppression for reflux disease: "off-the-peg" or a tailored approach? Clin Gastroenterol Hepatol. 2012;10:210.
13. Gill SK, O'Brien L, Einarson TR, Koren G. The safety of proton pump inhibitors (PPIs) in pregnancy: a meta-analysis. Am J Gastroenterol. 2009;104:1541.
14. Ip S, Chung M, Moorthy D, Yu WW, Lee J, Chan JA, et al. Comparative effectiveness of management strategies for gastroesophageal reflux disease: update. Rockville: Agency for Healthcare Research and Quality (US); 2011. Report No. 11-EHC049-EF
15. Behm BW, Peura DA. Dexlansoprazole MR for the management of gastroesophageal reflux disease. Expert Rev Gastroenterol Hepatol. 2011;5(4):439–45.
16. De Giorgi F, Savarese MF, Atteo E, Leone CA, Cuomo R. Medical treatment of gastro-oesophageal reflux disease. Acta Otorhinolaryngol Ital. 2006;26(5):276–80.

17. Wolfe MM, Sachs G. Acid suppression; optimizing therapy for gastroduodenal ulcer healing, gastroesophageal reflux disease, and stress-related erosive syndrome. Gastroenterology. 2000;118:S9.
18. Tytgat GN, Nio CY. The medical therapy of reflux oesophagitis. Baillieres Clin Gastroenterol. 1987;1(4):791–807.
19. Fock KM, Talley NJ, Fass R, Goh KL, Katelaris P, Hunt R, et al. Asia-Pacific consensus on the management of gastroesophageal reflux disease: update. Gastroenterol Hepatol. 2008;23:8–22.
20. Sontag SJ. The medical management of reflux esophagitis. Role of antacids and acid inhibition. Gastroenterol Clin North Am. 1990;19:683.
21. Chiu CT, Hsu CM, Wang CC, Chang JJ, Sung CM, Lin CJ, et al. Randomised clinical trial: sodium alginate oral suspension is non-inferior to omeprazole in the treatment of patients with non-erosive gastroesophageal disease. Aliment Pharmacol Ther. 2013;38(9):1054–64.
22. Thomas E, Wade A, Crawford G, Jenner B, Levinson N, Wilkinson J. Randomised clinical trial: relief of upper gastrointestinal symptoms by an acid pocket-targeting alginate-antacid (Gaviscon double action) – a double-blind, placebo-controlled, pilot study in gastro-oesophageal reflux disease. Aliment Pharmacol Ther. 2014;39(6):595–602. Epub 2014 Jan 28
23. De Ruigh A, Roman S, Chen J, Pandolfino JE, Kahrilas PJ. Gaviscon double action liquid (antacid & alginate) is more effective than antacid in controlling post-prandial oesophageal acid exposure in GERD patients: a double-blind crossover study. Aliment Pharmacol Ther. 2014;40(5):531–7. Epub 2014 Jul 10
24. Ren LH, Chen WX, Qian LJ, Li S, Gu M, Shi RH. Addition of prokinetics to PPI therapy in gastroesophageal reflux disease: a meta-analysis. World J Gastroenterol. 2014;20(9):2412–9.
25. Champion MC. Prokinetic therapy in gastroesophageal reflux disease. Can J Gastroenterol. 1997;11(Suppl B):55B–65B.
26. Van Noord C, Dieleman JP, van Herpen G, Verhamme K, Sturkenboom MC. Domperidone and ventricular arrhythmia or sudden cardiac death: a population-based case-control study in the Netherlands. Drug Saf. 2010;33(11):1003–14.
27. Katz PO, Gerson LB, Vela MF. Diagnosis and management of gastroesophageal reflux disease. Am J Gastroenterol. 2013;108:308–28.
28. Liu Q, Feng CC, Wang EM, Yan XJ, Chen SL. Efficacy of mosapride plus proton pump inhibitors for treatment of gastroesophageal reflux disease: a systematic review. World J Gastroenterol. 2013;19(47):9111–8.
29. Tominaga K, Iwakiri R, Fujimoto K, Fujiwara Y, Tanaka M, Shimoyama Y, et al. Rikkunshito improves symptoms in PPI-refractory GERD patients: a prospective, randomized, multicenter trial in Japan. J Gastroenterol. 2012;47(3):284–92.
30. Yamane Y, Yamaguchi T, Tsumori M, Yamauchi M, Yano S, Yamamoto M, et al. Elcatonin is effective for lower back pain and the symptoms of gastroesophageal reflux disease in elderly osteoporotic patients with kyphosis. Geriatr Gerontol Int. 2011;11:215–20.
31. Dean B, Gano A Jr, Knight K, Ofman J, Fass R. Effectiveness of proton pump inhibitors in non-erosive reflux disease. Clin Gastroenterol Hepatol. 2004;2:654–64.
32. Ponce J, Arguello L, Bastida G, Ponce M, Ortiz V, Garrigues V. On-demand therapy with rabeprazole in nonerosive and erosive gastroesophageal reflux disease in clinical practice: effectiveness, health-related quality of life, and patient satisfaction. Dig Dis Sci. 2004;49:931–6.
33. Hughes D, Bodger K, Bytzer P, de Herdt D, Dubois D. Economic analysis of on-demand maintenance therapy with proton pump inhibitors in patients with non-erosive reflux disease. Pharmaeconomics. 2005;23:1031–41.
34. Wu JC, Chan FK, Ching JY, Leung WK, Lee YT, Sung JJ. Empirical treatment based on "typical" reflux symptoms is inappropriate in a population with a high prevalence of helicobacter pylori infection. Gastrointest Endosc. 2002;55(4):461–5.
35. Richter JE, Sabesin SM, Kogut DG, Kerr RM, Wruble LD, Collen MJ. Omeprazole versus ranitidine or ranitidine/metoclopramide in poorly responsive symptomatic gastroesophageal reflux disease. Am J Gastroenterol. 1996;91(9):1766–72.

36. Kiljander TO, Junghard O, Beckman O, Lind T. Effect of esomeprazole 40 mg once or twice daily on asthma: a randomized, placebo-controlled study. Am J Respir Crit Care Med. 2010;181(10):1042–8.
37. Harding SM, Sontag SJ. Asthma and gastroesophageal reflux. Am J Gastroenterol. 2000;95:S23–32.
38. Chan WW, Chiou E, Obstein KL, Tignor AS, Whitlock TL. The efficacy of proton pump inhibitors for the treatment of asthma in adults: a meta-analysis. Arch Intern Med. 2011;171(7):620–9.
39. Qadeer MA, Phillips CO, Lopez AR, Steward DL, Noordzij JP, Wo JM, et al. Proton pump inhibitor therapy for suspected GERD-related chronic laryngitis: a meta-analysis of randomized controlled trials. Am J Gastroenterol. 2006;101(11):2646–54.
40. Park W, Hicks D, Khandwala F, Richter JE, Abelson T, Milstein C, et al. Laryngeal reflux: prospective cohort study evaluating optimal dose of proton-pump inhibitor therapy and pretherapy predictors of response. Laryngoscope. 2005;115(7):1230–8.
41. Spechler SJ, Lee E, Ahnen D, Goyal RK, Hirano I, Ramirez F, et al. Long-term outcome of medical and surgical therapies for gastroesophageal reflux disease: follow-up of a randomized controlled trial. JAMA. 2001;285(18):2331–8.

Investigations and Treatment of PPI Refractory GERD

8

Kwong Ming Fock

Abstract

Gastroesophageal reflux disease (GERD) is a common gastrointestinal condition worldwide. Although not life threatening, it affects quality of life and health-care utilization. Most GERD patients are treated in primary care, until medical therapy fails, when a referral to a specialist, usually a gastroenterologist, occurs. Depending on the presenting symptoms and response to medical therapy, the causes of treatment failure can be GERD related or non-GERD related. Endoscopy, pH monitoring, and impedance pH monitoring are the investigations currently used for evaluation of proton pump inhibitor (PPI) refractory GERD. This review attempts to present an account of the current investigations, treatment, and the clinical context for which they are to be used.

Keywords

GERD • NERD • PPI therapy • Barrett's esophagus • PPI failure • Refractory GERD

Introduction

Gastroesophageal reflux disease (GERD) is a common condition affecting 10–20% of the population in the developed world and is increasingly common in Asia and other developing countries. Since their introduction for the treatment of GERD two decades ago, proton pump inhibitors (PPIs) have been shown in numerous clinical trials to be the most effective form of medical treatment. Most, if not all guidelines, recommend their use as the treatment of choice for GERD patients. PPIs are

K.M. Fock (✉)
Changi Hospital, National University of Singapore, Singapore, Singapore
e-mail: kwong_ming_fock@cgh.com.sg

© Springer India 2018
P. Sharma et al. (eds.), *The Rise of Acid Reflux in Asia*,
DOI 10.1007/978-81-322-0846-4_8

97

effective in symptom relief and healing of mucosal lesions. Despite their high degree of efficacy, failure in patient response to PPIs does occur. About 32% of patients diagnosed with GERD in primary care are reported to be refractory to PPIs. With the increasing use of PPIs as first-line therapy, PPI failure is expected to rise substantially. PPI failure has become a common clinical challenge for primary care providers and specialists.

In a post hoc analysis of the 2007 National Health and Wellness Survey (NHWS) carried out in the USA and Europe, GERD patients with persistent, intense symptoms despite proton pump therapy have a poorer health-related quality of life (HRQOL), lower work productivity, and higher absenteeism than patients with low symptom load. In addition, US respondents with persistent, intense symptoms reported more emergency room visits. A systematic review of 19 studies by Tack concluded disruptive GERD patients had 2.4 times higher mean rates of absenteeism, 1.5 times higher mean rates of presenteeism, 1.5 times lower sleep quality scores, and 1.3 times lower mean scores for psychological and general well-being. Thus, failure to respond to PPI in GERD patients impacts quality of life and increases health-care utilization.

Definition of PPI Failure (Refractory GERD)

There is currently no universally accepted definition of PPI failure. One proposed definition of PPI failure is 50% or less improvement in the chief complaint after at least 12 weeks of PPI therapy [1]. There are difficulties applying this definition in clinical practice, as this is patient-driven based on their expectations.

PPI Failure and GERD Phenotypes

GERD has been divided into three phenotypes by Fass [2]:

1. Nonerosive reflux disease (NERD) comprising 60–70% of GERD cases
2. Erosive esophagitis comprising 20–30%
3. Barrett's esophagus and other complications, about 6–10% of GERD

The Montreal definition and classification of GERD [3] added another group (very extraesophageal GERD syndromes) made up of conditions characterized by symptoms with established or proposed association with GERD. The exact prevalence of these syndromes is difficult to ascertain because the symptoms are nonspecific and the relationship with GERD requires investigations.

These three phenotypes of typical GERD exist separately and mostly remain in the same phenotype over time. Natural history studies demonstrate that 85–90% of NERD patients do not progress to develop erosive esophagitis or Barrett's esophagus. Likewise, patients with erosive esophagitis are unlikely to progress to Barrett's esophagus. Profiling the phenotype that contributes to the growing pool of PPI refractory, GERD patients will allow development of diagnostic techniques and therapy.

Reflux-Related Causes of PPI Failure
- Compliance
- Improper dosing
- Residual acid reflux
- Non-acid or weakly acidic reflux
- Acid pocket
- Duodenogastric reflux
- Esophageal hypersensitivity
- Concomitant functional disorder including overlap syndromes
- Psychological comorbidity
- Nocturnal acid breakthrough
- PPI metabolism and CYP2C19 polymorphism

Erosive Esophagitis and PPI Failure

Clinical studies in patients with erosive esophagitis have demonstrated 88–96% [4] healing rates following 8 weeks of PPI therapy. Despite healing of mucosal lesions, up to 15% of patients with erosive esophagitis continue to experience GERD symptoms. Erosive esophagitis constitutes less than 30% of patients, who are PPI refractory.

Barrett's Esophagus and PPI Failure

The prevalence of Barrett's esophagus is 6–12% of all GERD patients [4] who are endoscoped and about 0.25–3.9% in all patients undergoing upper GI endoscopy. Symptom relief in patients with Barrett's esophagus is about 80%, although abnormal acid exposure can be demonstrated in 20–40% of patients. With higher-dose PPIs, complete heartburn resolution occurs symptomatic in 80–85% [4] of patients with Barrett's esophagus; thus, 15–20% of patients with Barrett's esophagus are refractory to PPI.

Nonerosive Reflux Disease (NERD) and PPI Failure

As 70% of patients with typical symptoms in a primary care setting do not have mucosal injury, they are diagnosed as NERD. In a systematic review of the literature, PPI symptom response pooled rate was as low as 36.7% in NERD [4] patients. Therefore, most of the PPI refractory patients are likely to come from NERD. It has been shown that esophageal acid exposure and symptoms resolution are directly related. The greater the esophageal acid exposure, the higher the response rate. Thus it is useful to subdivide NERD patients according to the esophageal acid exposure and their response to PPI. The subtypes are:

1. *Nonerosive reflux disease (NERD)*. These patients have normal endoscopy but abnormal esophageal acid exposure on pH studies. The response to standard dose of PPI is better than the other two subtypes described below.
2. *Hypersensitive esophagus*. At endoscopy these patients have normal endoscopy, normal acid exposure on pH monitoring, but positive symptom-reflux association (symptom index: SI > 50%, SAP > 95%). These patients have a limited response to standard-dose PPIs but show improvement when higher doses are used.
3. *Functional heartburn*. These patients have at endoscopy normal endoscopy mucosa, normal acid exposure, and negative symptom-reflux association. They rarely respond to PPIs.

Non-cardiac Chest Pain (NCCP) and PPI Failure

In the Montreal classification of GERD, non-cardiac chest pain was classified under symptomatic esophageal syndrome. The response of NCCP to PPI was reported in 68 studies, [5] of which three studies were double-blind, placebo controlled involving treatment with PPIs for 4–8 weeks. Two studies showed significant response to PPI (81%, 33%), and the placebo response rate was 6% and 25%, respectively. PPI refractory NCCP could be an important clinical issue in some regions.

Extraesophageal Syndromes and PPI Failure

The Montreal classification introduced the concept of extraesophageal syndromes that have an established or a proposed association with GERD. Although there are epidemiologic and physiologic evidence for an association, there is insufficient evidence to show causality. The extraesophageal syndromes are (1) reflux cough syndrome, (2) reflux laryngitis syndrome, (3) reflux asthma syndrome, and (4) dental erosion syndrome. A therapeutic benefit for acid-suppressive therapy in patients with extraesophageal syndromes such as chronic cough could not be dismissed, but evidence suggests that rigorous patient selection is required to identify patients most likely to respond [6]. The proportion of patients with extraesophageal syndromes who are refractory to PPI is not well documented.

Mechanisms of PPI Failure

Broadly speaking, the factors that could contribute to GERD symptoms despite PPI therapy would fall into two categories:

1. Non-reflux-related causes
2. Reflux-related causes

Non-reflux-Related Causes of PPI Failure

The non-reflux-related causes of refractory GERD include esophageal motility disorders such as impaired gastric emptying and outlet obstruction due to pyloric stenosis or gastric tumor.

Pill esophagitis is caused by medicinal pills that dissolve in the esophagus rather than passing rapidly into the stomach. Common drugs that cause pill esophagitis are antibiotics—especially the newer tetracyclines—bisphosphonates, iron supplements, NSAIDs, and aspirin. Patients with eosinophilic esophagitis usually present with dysphagia, with only about one-third of patients reporting typical heartburn. Prevalence of eosinophilic esophagitis in patients with heartburn ranged between 0.9 and 8.8%. At endoscopy, ridges, farrows, rings, or even multiple rings can be seen. Presence of white exudates is suggestive of eosinophilic esophagitis. Histologically, eosinophilic inflammation is present. At least 15 eosinophils per high-power field are required for diagnosis. Patients with eosinophilic esophagitis may respond to PPIs [7].

> **Non-reflux-Related Causes of PPI Failure**
> 1. Esophageal motility disorders: e.g., achalasia, scleroderma
> 2. Other non-reflux-related esophagitis: pill esophagitis, eosinophilic esophagitis, and infectious esophagitis
> 3. Functional chest pain
> 4. Functional heartburn
> 5. Other causes of chronic cough hoarseness
> 6. Impaired gastric emptying

Functional Heartburn

Functional heartburn is a diagnosis by exclusion based on functional testing and normal endoscopy. It is a distinct entity from NERD and is a common cause for PPI failure in patients with reflux symptoms. Using impedance pH monitoring and a dyspepsia questionnaire, a study demonstrated that there was an increased prevalence of dyspeptic symptoms in patients with functional heartburn and suggested that functional heartburn has more in common with functional dyspepsia than with NERD [8].

Reflux-Related Causes of PPI Failure

Compliance and Improper Dosing

Poor compliance is common in patients with GERD. After 1 month of therapy, only about 55% of GERD patients continued their PPI as instructed by their physician [9]. PPIs should be taken 30 min before breakfast and dinner to achieve maximum acid inhibition. Patients, however, take PPIs incorrectly, and a study found 39% of patients took the PPI at bedtime instead. There is no direct evidence that strict adherence to dosing schedule can improve symptoms.

Residual Acid Reflux

Residual acid reflux has been demonstrated in patients with persistent heartburn despite taking PPIs once or twice daily. In a recent study, Karamanolis demonstrated that 16% and 32% of symptomatic patients on double-dose and standard-dose PPIs, respectively, have abnormal pH tests [10]. Positive symptom index (SI) with an acid reflux event was seen in 40% of patients who were deemed PPI failures on PPIs once daily [11].

Weakly Acidic or Non-acid Reflux

Non-acid gastroesophageal reflux refers to refluxates with pH > 4 and was demonstrated on multichannel intraluminal impedance (MII) with pH sensor. The first postprandial impedance pH study in patients on PPI twice daily documented most of the reflux events were non-acidic. Non-acidic reflux was associated with typical heartburn, although less often than acidic reflux. Other symptoms such as regurgitation and sour or bitter taste in mouth were also associated with non-acid reflux.

Acid Pocket

Non-acid reflux episodes and heartburn occur during the postprandial period. This observation appears contradictory, as intragastric pH is highest (least acidic), following a meal due to the buffering effect of food. In 2001, Fletcher carried out a series of experiments using stepwise pull-through of a pH electrode from proximal stomach into the esophagus in healthy volunteers after a high-fat meal. The investigation detected an area of unbuffered, highly acidic gastric juice at the esophago-gastric junction that escapes the buffering effect of a meal. This area of high activity detected in the proximal stomach after a meal is termed acid pocket. Acid pocket can be found in healthy patients as well as in GERD patients and serves as a reservoir for acid reflux. In GERD patients, the acid pocket has a tendency toward upward migration. In the presence of a hiatus hernia, the acid pocket is in a supradiaphragmatic position, and the propensity for acid reflux is further increased. A recent study demonstrated that after PPI treatment, the acid pocket remained but became smaller and less acidic, and pH increased from 1 to 4. Further research into the acid pocket would be needed to elucidate its role in PPI refractory GERD.

Esophageal Hypersensitivity

Patients with persistent reflux symptoms despite PPI therapy may have normal esophagus acid exposure and normal endoscopy but a positive correlation between symptoms and acid and non-acid reflux events. This is analogous to the visceral hyperalgesia that is seen in other functional gastrointestinal disorders.

Nocturnal Acid Breakthrough (NAB)

Nocturnal acid breakthrough was initially proposed as a major cause of refractory GERD. However, later studies have shown that 70% of patients with refractory GERD experienced NAB, but only in 36% was there a correlation between reflux symptoms and NAB.

Bile Acid Reflux

Early studies suggested that 10–15% of non-acid reflux could be caused by bile reflux. More recent studies, however, demonstrate that most bile reflux occurred with acid reflux, and acid suppression does not guarantee elimination of bile reflux. In a study that included 65 patients with persistent reflux symptoms while on PPI, a number of bile reflux events and symptoms were correlated, suggesting a role for bile reflux.

Impaired Gastric Emptying

Patients who have impaired gastric emptying are predisposed to reflux. Examples are peptic ulcer or gastric tumor causing gastric outlet obstruction.

Psychological Comorbidity

Patients with GERD demonstrate significantly higher anxiety and depression scores when compared with normal subjects. Psychological comorbidity in GERD has been shown to predict the occurrence of GERD-related symptoms regardless of mucosal injury. In our own study in Asia, we found a significantly higher prevalence of minor psychiatric comorbidities in NERD patients (46.7%) and patients with erosive esophagitis (26.4%) compared with 16.8% in the general population [12]. Patients with non-cardiac chest pain, nutcracker esophagus show a tendency to be hypochondriac and seek medical care early. Thus psychological comorbidity is common among GERD patients and appears to affect all GERD phenotypes. Some patients with GERD do report that their reflux symptoms are triggered by or aggravated during stressful periods.

Concomitant Functional Gastrointestinal Disease

Patients with GERD frequently report dyspeptic symptoms such as nausea, vomiting, early satiety, bloating, and belching. In a recent systematic review, it was found that 38% of GERD patients have dyspeptic symptoms [13]. Patients with NERD had a higher percentage of dyspeptic symptoms compared with erosive GERD patients and had a lower response rate of response with PPIs. This group of patients will require treatment for dyspepsia. Another recent study reported that functional dyspepsia and irritable bowel syndrome are strongly associated with PPI failure in patients with GERD diagnosed on impedance pH studies.

Diagnostic Evaluation

History and Physical Examination

1. Check for non-GERD-related causes, particularly in extraesophageal syndrome.
2. Check drug history for pill esophagitis and other non-GERD-related causes, and check body weight and BMI.
3. Differentiate from functional disorders. The bothersome symptom(s) that is persistent despite PPI therapy should be carefully evaluated. Epigastric burning and heartburn are two symptoms which can be misinterpreted. Epigastric burning is, according to Rome III definition, a feature of dyspepsia and does not have a cephalad retrosternal radiation. By careful history taking, it is possible to detect functional GI disorders. Check for alarm symptoms.
4. Symptoms such as dysphagia, odynophagia, weight loss, anorexia, or upper GI bleeding are red flags for structural disorders. On the other hand, the absence of alarm symptoms should not lead the clinician to complacency.
5. Check the time that the persistent troublesome symptoms occur. This information will help to determine if nocturnal acid breakthrough or acid pocket could be the mechanism for PPI failure.
6. Check for proper dosing and correct timing of PPIs. This should be done before embarking on further investigations and can be improved through patient education.
7. Check for psychological morbidity. Stress can aggravate reflux symptoms and negatively affect the response to PPI.

In patients without alarm symptoms, increasing the dose of a PPI or switching to a different PPI before initiating diagnostic testing can be considered. A randomized controlled trial in patients with persistent GERD symptoms taking a single daily dose of PPI showed that increasing PPI to twice daily or switching to another PPI resulted in symptomatic improvement in about 20% of patients.

Upper GI Endoscopy

Patients who fail to respond either completely or partially to PPIs despite optimization of PPI therapy require further diagnostic workup. Those with typical esophageal symptoms should undergo endoscopy.

When an upper GI endoscopy and biopsy are performed, there is some evidence that dilated intercellular spaces (DIS) may help to differentiate NERD from functional heartburn. Our group has also reported usefulness of narrowband imaging to diagnose GERD [14]. In patients suspected of suffering from eosinophilic esophagitis, esophageal biopsy should be obtained. Obtaining esophageal biopsy in patients with refractory GERD to diagnose eosinophilic esophagitis is cost-effective only when the prevalence of eosinophilic esophagitis is more than 8%, according to a Markov model analysis [15].

An observational study was performed to compare the endoscopic findings in patients who failed to obtain complete or partial response to 8 weeks of once-daily PPI treatment versus patients with reflux symptoms who received no treatment. GERD-related findings were significantly less common in the PPI-treated group compared with those who had not received treatment. Barrett's esophagus was found in about 3% of patients in both groups. Non-GERD-related findings were eosinophilic esophagitis (0.9%), achalasia (0.95%), gastric ulcer (0.95%), gastric/duodenal polyps (10.5% vs 6.6%), gastric cancer (0, 1.1%), and duodenal ulcer (0, 3.3%) [16]. This study demonstrated that upper GI endoscopy has a low diagnostic yield in PPI refractory patients.

Reflux Monitoring

Patients with PPI refractory reflux symptoms and normal endoscopy (NERD) should undergo further investigations, including 24 h pH monitoring and impedance testing. Patients with extraesophageal syndromes after exclusion of non-GERD-related etiology for their symptoms should be considered for reflux monitoring.

Currently, available tests for reflux monitoring are (1) catheter pH monitoring, (2) wireless pH, (3) combined multichannel pH monitor, and (4) esophageal Bilitec monitoring. Each technique has its limitations. Twenty-four hour pH monitoring has a sensitivity of 70–80% in typical GERD syndromes and the false negative rate ranges from 20 to 50%. With extraesophageal syndromes, the sensitivity is lower than with esophageal syndromes (50%). Day-to-day variation in acid exposure is an important reason for the high false negative rate. By extending pH monitoring to 48 or 96 h, a wireless ambulatory pH capsule can improve the diagnostic yield. In PPI refractory patients with negative catheter-based pH studies, our experience with Bravo is that it led to an increased diagnostic yield of 30% [17].

Charbel found that 31% of patients with typical symptoms and 30% of those with extraesophageal symptoms have abnormal pH testing (catheter based) [18] when treated with once-daily PPI, while with twice-daily PPI only 7% and 1%, respectively, had an abnormal pH test. The results suggested that once-daily PPI is insufficient to inhibit acid, and by increasing the dose, acidic reflux is no longer the main cause of patient's symptoms. Rather, non-acid reflux (NAR) is the main driver for patient's symptoms. Impedance pH study is the technique for detection of non-acid reflux, which can be liquid, gas, or mixture of both.

When a decision is made for reflux monitoring, two key issues need to be resolved: (1) what technique to use and (2) whether PPI therapy should be stopped for reflux monitoring. The technique chosen depends on the patient's clinical presentation (esophageal or extraesophageal) as well as the available technology and expertise. Reflux monitoring "off PPI" as well as "on PPI" offers clinically useful information, although there is no general agreement on which test has a higher diagnostic yield.

Reflux monitoring "off PPI" (7 days after cessation of PPI) can be performed using any of the available techniques described above. A negative test (normal esophageal acid exposure and negative symptom-reflux association) means that the patient is most likely to be suffering from functional heartburn [19]. Rome III definition of functional heartburn reflux refers only to 24 h pH monitoring, but the added value of impedance has to be considered, as non-acid reflux can be detected and therefore would reduce the proportion of functional heartburn (29% vs. 39% with 24 h pH only).

Reflux monitoring "on PPI" should be performed with impedance pH monitoring to allow detection of non-acid reflux [19]. The diagnostic yield with techniques other than impedance is very low, as in most acid-suppressed patients reflux is mainly non-acidic or usually acidic. It is not known whether wireless pH monitoring allowing both "off" and "on" PPI assessments could be more useful. Several reports have been published on the diagnosis made with PPI refractory patients tested with pH impedance: 50–60% of patients are non-GERD, 30–40% are caused by non-acid reflux, and 10% are due to acid reflux [20, 21]. Although uncommon, a positive test for acid reflux is evidence of therapeutic failure of GERD.

Studies comparing the yield of "on" and "off" PPI reflux monitoring are limited. A technical review on this issue suggested that the decision may be made based on the patient's clinical presentation. In patients with extraesophageal symptoms and without concomitant typical GERD symptoms, pH monitoring off medication may be more useful, as it will exclude GERD. In patients who have typical symptoms and partial response to PPI, it may be better off having reflux monitoring performed with PPI, as it would be possible to detect ongoing reflux due to therapeutic failure or noncompliance. For patients suspected of functional heartburn, off-therapy monitoring is preferred.

Another controversial issue is clinical value of SI or SAP. Slaughter et al. have shown that SI and SAP values were largely determined by chance occurrences [22]. Nonetheless, despite the shortcomings, analyses of symptom-reflux association are still clinically helpful to improve diagnosis of GERD-related symptoms.

Bilitec esophageal monitoring does not appear to be a first choice for diagnosis evaluation in PPI refractory patients, as the diagnostic yield is low and availability is limited.

Treatment of Refractory GERD

Optimizing PPI Treatment

The first step in the management of refractory is to optimize PPI therapy by checking compliance and confirming correct dosing, especially the evening dose rather than at bedtime.

Treatment of Residual Acid Reflux

After establishing compliance and correct dosing, increasing PPI to twice-daily dose or switching to another PPI could result in systematic improvement in roughly 20% of patients. There is no evidence to support further increase of PPI in those who failed PPI twice daily.

Lifestyle Modifications

Although lifestyle modifications such as weight loss and elevation of the head of the bed form part of the therapy for GERD, their value in refractory GERD patients has yet to be demonstrated. Recently, training the diaphragm by means of breathing exercises has been shown to improve GERD as assessed by pH study, quality of life, and PPI usage. There is no study to date that has shown clinical improvement in GERD symptoms by excluding coffee, chocolate, syrup, or fatty or spicy food [19].

Treatment Targeted at Residual Acidic Reflux

Based on the observation that 75% of patients taking PPI twice daily exhibit nocturnal acid breakthrough, H2RAs have been added at bedtime for patients with refractory GERD. Nocturnal acid control has been shown to improve. But there is a paucity of clinical data to show symptom improvement. Furthermore, patients taking H2RAs develop tachyphylaxis, and therefore most practitioners who use H2RAs use it intermittently or on demand.

Transient lower esophageal sphincter relaxations (TLESRs) are the main mechanism of all types of reflux—acidic, weakly acidic, or non-acidic. Currently, the only medication that can decrease TLESRs is baclofen, a $GABA_B$ agonist. Two studies have shown that baclofen can improve reflux-related symptoms [23, 24]. Baclofen use has been limited by CNS adverse effects. Many patients report dizziness, drowsiness, nausea, and vomiting. Newer $GABA_B$ agonists such as arbaclofen placarbil and lesogaberan have better tolerability but reduced efficacy.

Treatment Used for Gastroesophageal Motility

Prokinetic therapy with metoclopramide in addition to PPI is another option for patients with refractory GERD. Metoclopramide has been shown to increase lower esophageal sphincter pressure and accelerate gastric emptying. Domperidone is a peripherally acting dopamine agonist that has been demonstrated to improve gastric emptying too, but there is a paucity of data supporting its use in GERD. Metoclopramide has CNS side effects and in <1% of patients causes tardive dyskinesia. Checking for QT prolongation before starting domperidone may be prudent, as there is a small risk of ventricular arrhythmia.

Mosapride, a $5HT_4$ receptor agonist and weak $5HT_4$ receptor antagonist, has been shown to reduce acid reflux in the esophagus by improving esophageal motility and gastric emptying. In a study investigating efficacy with mosapride as an add-on therapy with omeprazole in PPI-resistant NERD patients, reflux symptoms and gastric emptying were shown to improve in a subset of patients with delayed gastric emptying. Itopride, a dopamine 2 agonist, has been used in patients as an acid or with PPIs for laryngopharyngeal reflux. Compared to placebo it has a faster improvement rate, but not greater efficacy. Rikkunshito, a traditional Japanese medicine, has been used in combination with PPI in patients with refractory GERD [25].

Targeting the Acid Pocket

A new target for treatment of reflux, and possibly refractory GERD, is the acid pocket. In the presence of a hiatus hernia, the acid pocket was more frequently located within the hiatus above the diaphragm, leading to increased acid reflux. In a pilot study, an alginate-antacid formulation has been recently demonstrated to reduce the number of acid reflux episodes by displacing the acid pocket below the diaphragm in patients with symptomatic GERD and large hiatus hernia. Confirmatory studies with larger number of patients will be needed before the alginate-antacid becomes standard therapy.

Treatment of Esophageal Hypersensitivity

Most patients with GERD symptoms refractory to PPI have normal esophageal acid exposure and normal endoscopy. On pH testing, they could have positive or negative symptom-reflux association. The latter group fulfills the criteria of functional heartburn (Rome III criteria), while the former group has been labeled as hypersensitive esophagus. In both groups, visceral hypersensitivity has a role. Pain modulators such as tricyclic antidepressants (TCAs), trazodone, and selective serotonin reuptake inhibitors (SSRIs) have all been shown to improve esophageal pain in patients with non-cardiac chest pain. According to current understanding, these agonists confer their visceral analgesic effect by acting at the central nervous system and/or afferent levels. The doses used are small and do not alter moods. For patients who have refractory heartburn and do not have access to esophageal impedance pH testing, a trial of one of these medications is an alternative. Other compounds that may potentially exert an influence on visceral hypersensitivity include citalopram, A_2D1386, and tegaserod. Further evaluation of these drugs is needed.

Endoscopic Therapy

Although short-term results with endoscopic devices have been encouraging, long-term efficacy has been elusive. A recent report of LINX reflux system made of titanium beads shows efficacy up to 4 years with few side effects in a multicenter trial and has obtained FDA approval [26].

Surgical Treatment

Laparoscopic fundoplication is effective in controlling acid and non-acid reflux. A recent randomized controlled study demonstrated that in PPI-responsive patients, esomeprazole and anti-reflux surgery achieved comparable rates of remission at 5 years. However, there is controversy on the efficacy of anti-reflux surgery in patients who have normal endoscopy and normal/abnormal acid exposure. It is prudent at this time to limit anti-reflux surgery to patients who are refractory to PPI and who have abnormal acid exposure when tested "off PPI."

Management algorithm of patients with PPI refractory symptom is shown in Fig. 8.1.

Conclusion

The advent of acid-suppressive drugs, in particular proton pump inhibitors (PPI), has revolutionized the management of GERD, with the promise that GERD could soon be a disease of the past. However, although many patients respond to PPI, refractory GERD has emerged as the new clinical challenge. Most, if not all, of

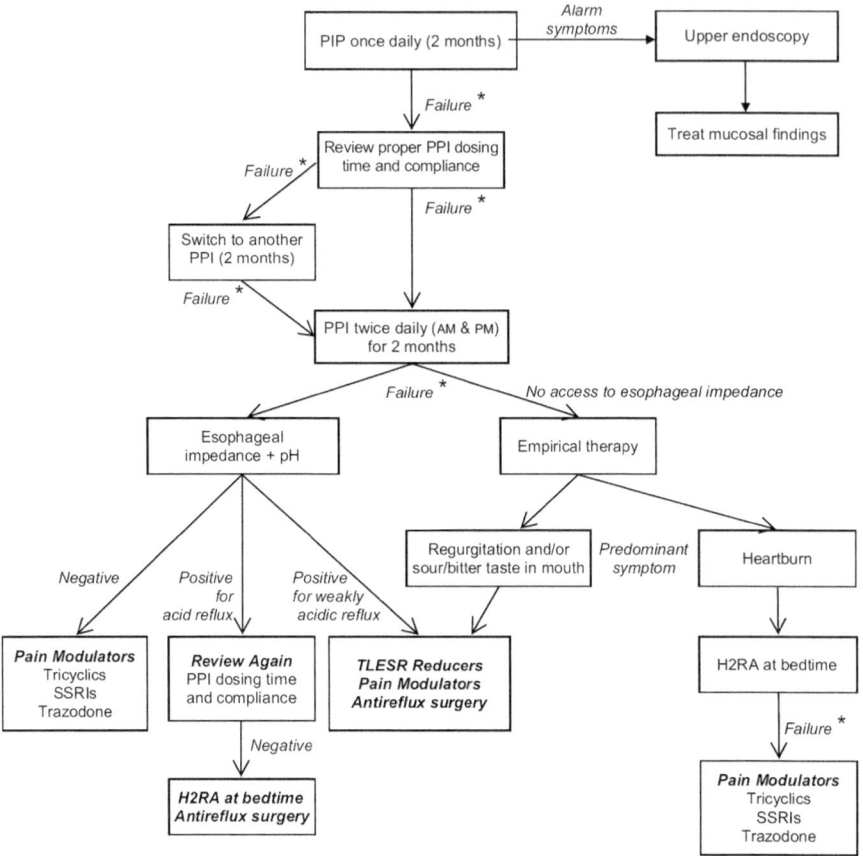

Fig. 8.1 Management algorithm of patients with PPI refractory symptom (Reprinted from Best Pract Res Clin Gastroenterol, Dec;24(6):923–36; Hershcovici T, Fass R. An algorithm for diagnosis and treatment of refractory GERD; © 2010, with permission from Elsevier)

these patients refractory to PPI are NERD and the extraesophageal syndromes. The reasons for their failure to respond to treatment are due to GERD-related or non-GERD-related etiologies. Currently, technologies to better measure pH and acid exposure in the esophagus have been developed to distinguish the PPI refractory GERD patients from non-GERD patients. It remains to be seen if the outcomes of treatment match the proposed mechanisms of PPI refractories.

References

1. Stifim D, Zebib F. Diagnosis and management of patients with reflux symptoms refractory to proton pump inhibitors. Gut. 2012;61:1340–54.
2. Fass R, Ofman JJ. Gastroesophageal reflux disease – should we adopt a new conceptual framework? Am J Gastroenterol. 2002;97:1901–9.

3. Vakil N, Van Zanten SV, Kahrilas P, Dent J, Jones R. Global consensus group. The Montreal definition and classification of gastroesophageal reflux disease: a global evidence-based consensus. Am J Gastroenterol. 2006;101(8):1900–20. quiz 1943

4. Fass R, Shapiro M, Dekel R, Sewell J. Systematic review: proton pump inhibitor failure in gastro-esophageal reflux disease – what next? Aliment Pharmacol Ther. 2005;22:79–94.

5. Hershcovici T, Archem SR, Jha LK, Fass R. Systematic review: the treatment of non-cardiac chest pain aliment. Pharmacol Ther. 2012;35:5–14.

6. Kahrilas PJ, Howden CW, Hughes N, Molloy-Bland M. Response of chronic cough to acid suppressive therapy in patients with gastroesophageal reflux disease. Chest. 2013;143:605–12.

7. Dellon ES, Gonsalves N, Hirano I, Furuta GT, Liacouras CA, Katzka DA, et al. ACG clinical guidelines: evidence based approach to the diagnosis and management of esophageal eosinophilia and eosinophilic esophagitis (EoE). Am J Gastroenterol. 2013;108:379–92.

8. Savarino E, Pohl D, Zentilin P, Dulbecco P, Sanmito G, Sconfienza L, et al. Functional heartburn has more in common with functional dyspepsia than with non-erosive reflux disease. Gut. 2009;58(9):1185–91.

9. The Gallop Organisation. Gallop Study of Consumers' use of stomach relief products. Princeton: The Gallop Organisation; 2000.

10. Karamanolis G, Vanuystel T, Sifrin D, Bisschops R, Arts J, Caenepeel P, et al. Yield of 24-hour esophageal pH and Bilitec monitoring in patients with persisting symptoms on PPI therapy. Dig Dis Sci. 2008;53:2387–93.

11. Kahrilas PJ, McColl K, Fox M, O'Rourke L, Sifrim D, Smout AJ, et al. The acid pocket: a target for treatment in reflux disease? Am J Gastroenterol. 2013;108:1058–64.

12. Ang TL, Fock KM, Ng TM, Teo EK, Chua TS, Tan J. A comparison of the clinical demographic and psychiatric profiles among patients with erosive and non-erosive reflex disease in a multi-ethnic Asian country. World J Gastroenterol. 2009;11:3558–61.

13. Gerson LB, Kahrilas PJ, Fass R. Insights into gastroesophageal reflux disease – associated dyspeptic symptoms. Clin Gastroenterol Hepatol. 2007;5:690–5.

14. Fock KM, Teo EK, Ang TL, Tan JY, Lam NM. The utility of narrow based imaging in improving the endoscopic diagnosis of gastroesophageal reflux disease. Clin Gastroenterol Hepatol. 2009;7:54–9.

15. Miller SM, Goldstein JL, Gerson LB. Cost effectiveness model of endoscopic biopsy for eosinophilia esophagitis in patients with refractory GERD. Am J Gastroenterol. 2011;106:1439–45.

16. Poh CH, Gasiorowska A, Navaro-Rodriguez J, Willis MR, Hargadon D, Noelck N, et al. Upper GI tract findings in patients with heartburn in whom proton pump inhibitor treatment failed versus those not receiving antireflux treatment. Gastrointest Endosc. 2010;71:28–34.

17. Ang D, Teo EK, Ang TL, Ong J, Poh CH, Tan J, et al. To Bravo or not? A comparison of wireless esophageal pH monitoring and conventional pH catheter to evaluate non-erosive gastroesophageal reflux disease in a multiracial Asian cohort. J Dig Dis. 2010;11:19–27.

18. Charbel S, Khandwala F, Vaezi MF. The role of esophageal pH monitoring in symptomatic patients as PPI therapy. Am J Gastroenterol. 2005;100:283–9.

19. Katz PO, Gerson LB, Vela MF. Guidelines for diagnosis and management of gastroesophageal reflux disease. Am J Gastroenterol. 2001;108:308–28.

20. Mainie I, Tutuian R, Shays S, Vela M, Zhang X, Sifrim D, et al. Acid and non-acid reflux in patients with persistent symptoms despite acid suppressive therapy: a multicenter study using combined ambulatory impedance-pH monitoring. Gut. 2006;55:1398–402.

21. Zerbib F, Roman S, Ropert A, des Varannes SB, Pouderoux P, Chaput U, et al. Esophageal pH-impedance monitoring and symptom analysis in GERD: a study in patients off and on therapy. Am J Gastroenterol. 2006;101:1956–63.

22. Slaughter JC, Goutte M, Rymer JA, , Oranu AC, Schneider JA, Garrett CG, et al. Caution about over interpretation of symptom indexes in reflux monitoring for refractory gastroesophageal reflux disease. Clin Gastroenterol Hepatol 2011;9:868–874.

23. Koek GH, Sifrim D, Lerut T, Janssens J, Tack J. Effect of the GABA(B) agonist baclofen in patients with symptoms and duodeno-gastro-oesophageal reflux refractory to proton pump inhibitors. Gut. 2003;52:1397–402.

24. Cossentino MJ, Mann K, Armbruster SP, Lake JM, Maydonovitch C, Wong RK. Randomised clinical trial: the effect of baclofen in patients with gastro-oesophageal reflux–a randomised prospective study. Aliment Pharmacol Ther. 2012;35:1036–44.
25. Tominaga K, Iwakiri R, Fujimoto K, Fujiwara Y, Tanaka M, Shimoyama Y, et al. Rikkunshito improves symptoms in PPI-refractory GERD patients: a prospective, randomized, multicenter trial in Japan. J Gastroenterol. 2012;47:284–92.
26. Ganz RA, Peters JH, Horgan S, Bemelman WA, Dunst CM, Edmundowicz SA, et al. Esophageal sphincter device for gastroesophageal reflux disease. N Engl J Med. 2013;368:719–27.

Surgical Treatment for Gastroesophageal Reflux Disease (GERD) in Asia

9

Sally Wai Yin Luk and Philip W.Y. Chiu

Abstract

The incidence of gastroesophageal reflux disease (GERD) is increasing in Asia. The majority of the patients are treated by long-term usage of proton pump inhibitors (PPI). Anti-reflux surgery had been considered as an equivalent alterative to long-term PPI. However, few studies have investigated the performance of anti-reflux surgery for the treatment of GERD in Asia. In this chapter, we review the current evidence and application of anti-reflux surgery for the treatment of GERD in Asia.

Keywords

Gastroesophageal reflux disease • Anti-reflux surgery • Laparoscopic fundoplication

Introduction

Gastroesophageal reflux disease (GERD) is a disorder in which duodenogastric contents reflux recurrently into the esophagus, causing troublesome symptoms and/or complications [1, 2]. From the surgical perspective, this is the failure of the anti-reflux flap valve mechanism at the esophagogastric junction (OGJ) that allows the

S.W.Y. Luk • P.W.Y. Chiu (✉)

Division of Upper GI and Metabolic Surgery, Department of Surgery, Institute of Digestive Disease, The Chinese University of Hong Kong, Hong Kong SAR, China

e-mail: philipchiu@surgery.cuhk.edu.hk

© Springer India 2018

P. Sharma et al. (eds.), *The Rise of Acid Reflux in Asia*,

DOI 10.1007/978-81-322-0846-4_9

backflow of gastric contents into the esophagus [3]. The symptoms are considered to be troublesome when they adversely affect one's quality of life (QOL) [1].

While GERD has long been a public concern in the West [4], this is an emerging disease entity in Asian countries over the past two decades. According to population-based studies, prevalence of GERD in East Asia ranges from 2.5 to 7.8% [5], and, interestingly, it is much higher in West Asia, with reported prevalence up to 50% [6, 7]. It is estimated that GERD affects up to 5% of the Chinese population [8]. In Singapore, a population survey found more than a sixfold increase in reporting reflux symptoms in a cohort of 237 community residents, rising from 1.6% to 9.9% from 1994 to 1999 [9].

Another study from a Japanese center reported that prevalence of reflux esophagitis on endoscopic examination has increased from 0.8% in 1975 to 2.3% in 1997 [10]. The apparent rising trend could partly be due to the low awareness of the disease in the past, together with an aging population [11]. Apart from racial difference, Asians share similar risk factors for GERD as Caucasians do, including age, male sex, smoking, increasing BMI, family history, and higher socioeconomic status [11, 12]. The Westernization of lifestyle and worldwide epidemic of obesity could be the attributing factors for the increasing prevalence. [11] As a result, there is a need for more comprehensive management of GERD in the Asia-Pacific region.

Asia-Pacific consensus on the management of GERD was first published in 2004 and updated in 2008 [13, 14]. However, there is still a paucity of literature on the indications and the type of anti-reflux surgery (ARS) performed in the Asian population. In this chapter, we will overview challenges in the management of GERD, in particular the role of surgical intervention, in Asian countries.

Diagnostic Challenges

GERD has a spectrum of clinical presentations, encompassing at least three broad groups of patients presenting with: (a) typical reflux symptoms, including heartburn and/or acid reflux, but without reflux esophagitis, so-called nonerosive reflux disease (NERD); (b) atypical reflux symptoms; (c) erosive esophagitis, i.e., erosive reflux disease (ERD), with or without complications. The expression of heartburn is less clear in most of the Asian languages, leading to difficulty in making a correct clinical diagnosis, which often overlaps with symptoms of dyspepsia [15]. Moreover, it is not uncommon for Asian patients to have atypical manifestations, such as non-cardiac chest pain, as the sole presenting feature of GERD [16–18]. It is the clinicians' responsibility to clarify the terms, together with the awareness of the diagnosis, in the context of atypical symptoms. The 24-h ambulatory pH study is currently regarded as the most objective investigation to establish the diagnosis of GERD. In the Western literature, the determination of excessive acid exposure would depend on esophageal acid exposure time (percentage of pH < 4 at 5 cm from LES) of more than 5%, or a composite score >14.72 according to the revised Johnson-DeMeester score [19]. However, these criteria for excessive acid exposure have not been validated in the Asian population. Furthermore, owing to the relatively low prevalence of GERD in Asia, 24-h pH tests are usually limited to tertiary referral centers [14, 18].

It has been reported that up to 30% of patients with NERD have normal esophageal acid exposure time upon 24-h pH study [20, 21]. The exact pathophysiology in this subgroup is not well understood, yet the plausible visceral hypersensitivity to acid may play a role in causing symptoms [22].

Upper endoscopy has low sensitivity as an objective diagnostic tool, as a majority of Asian patients do not have reflux esophagitis, not to mention the presence of its associated complications such as peptic stricture or Barrett's esophagus [23]. In a study from Hong Kong, only 631 out of 16,606 patients had endoscopic evidence of esophagitis; 14 of those had stricture, and 10 had Barrett's esophagus [24]. Interestingly, the endoscopic definition of esophagogastric junction in Japan is according to distal end of esophageal palisade vessels instead of proximal extent of the gastric fold [25]. Coupled with the high performance of endoscopy in Japan, these may accountable for more prevalence of Barrett's esophagus among Japanese than in other Asian countries. Nonetheless, most published data in the literature has revealed the low prevalence of Barrett's esophagus in Asia ranging from 0.06 to 0.22% [26, 27]. With the high prevalence of *Helicobacter pylori* (*H. pylori*) in Asia, esophagogastroscopy is usually performed to rule out peptic ulcer disease and gastric cancer before embarking on management of GERD [14, 28, 29].

Challenges in Surgical Management

Most patients in Asia with GERD can be symptomatically controlled by proton pump inhibitors (PPI) [30, 31]. This is partly due to the smaller parietal cell mass in Asians and a high prevalence of *H. pylori* infection [32]. However, PPI only alleviates GERD symptoms, without tackling the underlying mechanical problem. The anti-reflux flap valve created after fundoplication aims at restoring the LES pressure. Moreover, anti-reflux surgery (ARS) abolished the trigger to transient lower esophageal sphincter relaxations (TLESRs) [33]. The recent concern regarding the long-term effect of PPIs in inducing osteoporotic fracture, infection, and altering pharmacokinetics of concomitant drugs like clopidogrel further enhances the role of surgery in managing GERD [34].

Indications for surgical intervention in Asia should follow international guidelines when the diagnosis of GERD is confirmed with objective evidence. These include those who (1) opt for surgery despite successful medical management, or (2) failed medical treatment, or (3) have complication of GERD, e.g., Barrett's esophagus and peptic strictures [35]. As response to PPI therapy tends to be better in Asian countries, few patients are referred for consideration of ARS. In our center, more than 80% of patients who underwent ARS were those who opted not for lifelong medication, while only 6% were having erosive esophagitis or Barrett's esophagus. As the average age for GERD occurrence ranged from 30 to 50 years, lifelong medication will pose a major impact on their quality of life and a significant burden of the medication cost.

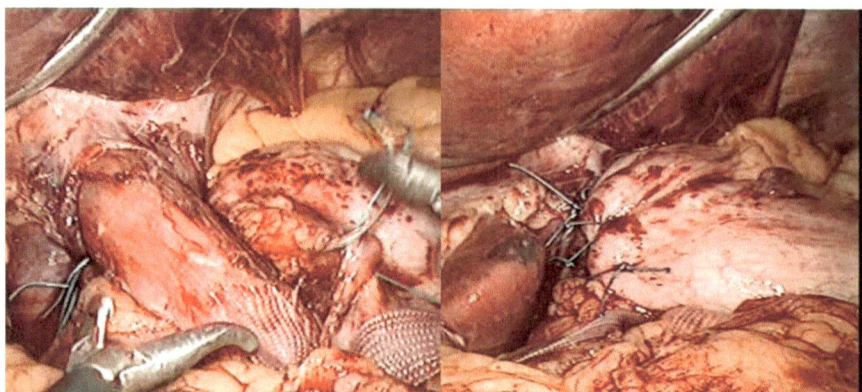

Fig. 9.1 Laparoscopic anterior partial fundoplication

Fig. 9.2 Laparoscopic
Nissen fundoplication

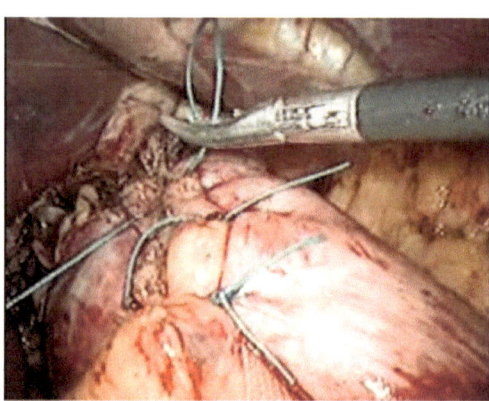

Since the introduction of anti-reflux surgery by Dr. Rudolf Nissen in 1954, fundoplication has become widely adopted as an alternative surgical treatment for GERD in the Caucasian population [36]. There has been development of different types of fundoplication, including Nissen 360 degree fundoplication and anterior and posterior partial fundoplication (Figs. 9.1 and 9.2). Up to the early 1990s, there were more than 12,000 open operations performed. With the advent of the first laparoscopic fundoplication by Dallemagne et al. in 1991 [37], the awareness of surgical treatment for GERD began to increase in Asia. The first report of laparoscopic fundoplication in an adult from Korea was published in 1996 [38]. In Hong Kong, our unit has performed laparoscopic anti-reflux procedures since the early 2000s. Subsequently, there were case series published from Japan, Korea, Malaysia, and India reporting the early surgical outcomes of the laparoscopic fundoplication in their countries [39–41].

Compared to Western countries, the development and performance of ARS have lagged behind in Asia due to low prevalence of GERD, surgical invasiveness compared to PPI, as well as patients' preference to medical therapy. Two meta-analyses published comparing clinical and perioperative outcomes of open versus laparoscopic ARS showed that laparoscopic ARS is associated with significant shorter hospital stay, with earlier return to normal activities, and less morbidity [42–44]. All the cohort studies from Asia had been using laparoscopic ARS (LARS) with 0% conversion rate, despite the fact that most Asian surgeons have limited experience in the open approach.

A recent randomized control trial from China by Cao et al. compared laparoscopic anterior 180-degree (LAF) versus Nissen fundoplication (LNF) [45]. This is the only clinical trial from Asia included in the meta-analysis comparing LAF versus LNF. This study included a select group of patient with erosive GERD and high DeMeester score. There were significantly fewer patients in the LAF group with dysphagia and gas-related symptoms at 5 years, which was consistent with the meta-analysis results. In general, there is a tendency favor toward LAF worldwide, including the Asia-Pacific region. On the other hand, there are still debates on some of the technical aspects that may influence surgical outcomes in the West; these include the division of short gastric vessels, crural repair, and the use of bougie to gauge the warp [46]. Division of short gastric vessels is usually recommended for the formation of short floppy Nissen fundoplication, and these vessels were preserved in anterior partial fundoplication. Though intraoperative placement of bougie is essential to prevent postoperative dysphagia, non-forceful insertion under direct vision with laparoscopy is essential to prevent perforation. Compared to studies in the West, where 56–58-Fr bougies were commonly used, the size of bougie is usually smaller for Asian patients, ranging from 46 to 50 Fr.

Surgical Outcome in Asia-Pacific Region

From the reported Asian case series in the literature, the early postoperative recovery was satisfactory. Most patients could start to have an oral fluid diet immediately after the operation and resume a soft diet on postoperative day 2. In our center, the mean hospital length of stays is 3.6 ± 1.5 days. Early postoperative complications ranged from 4 to 16% [39–44]. Major complications reported were esophageal perforation associated with the bougie insertion [44] and gastric perforation [39]. Most patients experienced some sort of side effect during the early postoperative period. These symptoms were temporary dysphagia, bloating, and increased flatulence, which would often improve with time. Temporary transient postoperative dysphagia was common, ranging from 35 to 40%. Persistent dysphagia requiring endoscopic dilatation was 9–16%, and the dysphagia rate was higher after Nissen fundoplication than partial.

Owing to the short-term follow-up of the case series, there was a paucity of reports concerning the long-term surgical outcomes, and most of the reports in the literature were retrospective cohorts. The only published prospective 5-year surgical outcome in Asia was from China by Cao et al. [44]. According to their results, at 5 years the dysphagia score was significantly higher in LNF than LAF. The results of our center were consistent with this randomized study, with more patients

Table 9.1 Clinical outcomes of a retrospective comparison between laparoscopic Nissen fundo-plication versus partial fundoplication at the Chinese University of Hong Kong

	LNF (39)	LPF (18)	P
Age	45.5	49.8	0.114
Gender (male:female)	25:14	13:5	
No of comorbidities	0.69	0.39	0.165
Esophagitis upon preoperative endoscopy	17 (43.6%)	11 (61.1%)	0.263
DeMeester score (preoperative)	21.1	39.6	0.07
Operative time (minutes)	129.8	152.7	0.114
Conversion	0	0	–
Hospital stay (days)	3.49	3.06	0.227
Reoperation	3 (7.7%)	1 (5.6%)	0.625
Recurrence of GERD	4 (10.5%)	5 (27.8%)	0.107
Dysphagia 4 weeks after surgery	11 (28.9%)	2 (11.1%)	0.126

LNF laparoscopic Nissen fundoplication; *LPF* laparoscopic partial fundoplication

developing dysphagia at the initial postoperative period after LNF. Out of the 60 patients who received LNF, 5 required endoscopic dilatation and subsequent redo fundoplication, while none of those after LAF developed persistent dysphagia.

Most studies defined recurrence of gastroesophageal reflux as need of redo fundoplication surgery or requirement of maintenance PPI. Recurrence of GERD 20–30 years was reported as 20–30% after open fundoplication, while recurrence at 5 years was around 5–15% for laparoscopic fundoplication [42]. The cause of recurrence was attributed to wrap disruption or migration. Cao et al. showed recurrence of GERD at 5 years was 15.63% (15 out of 96 patients, 8 in LAF, and 7 in LNF arms). Seven of them have undergone revision fundoplication, and GERD recurrence was confirmed with objective assessments including endoscopic examination and pH studies. Hence, laparoscopic fundoplication can achieve good reflux control among Chinese patients with erosive esophagitis. To note, the recurrence of reflux symptoms in Asian patients postoperatively needs particular attention, as this might not solely be caused by the recurrence of GERD. Owing to the high prevalence of *H. pylori* and risk of gastric cancer, further investigation including upper endoscopy is necessary prior to the prescription of maintenance PPI.

Our center conducted a retrospective comparison on the outcomes between laparoscopic Nissen fundoplication versus laparoscopic partial fundoplication in 57 patients in Hong Kong. There was no difference in the mean age and gender distribution between the two groups (Table 9.1). More than half of the patients who received fundoplication had endoscopic evidence of esophagitis (LNF group, 43.6%; LPF group, 61.1%; p = 0.263). There was no difference in the operative time between LNF and LPF. A total of four patients required reoperation, three in the LNF group and one in the LPF group. The reasons for reoperation in the LNF group were related to symptoms of dysphagia, while the reason for reoperation in the LPF group was due to recurrence of GERD. The overall rate of symptomatic control after laparoscopic fundoplication was 84.2%. There was a trend toward higher risks of symptom recurrence for laparoscopic partial fundoplication when compared to laparoscopic Nissen fundoplication, though not statistically significant.

Learning Curve and Training in Asian Countries

With the standardization of surgical techniques for LNF in Western countries [47], the acquisition of the skills becomes generally easier to follow for Asian surgeons who have limited experience in open fundoplication. Commonly, LNF is performed with the patient in lithotomy position and five-port technique—including two 10 mm ports and three 5 mm ports with one of them tailored for liver retraction. The learning curve was well documented in the literature, reporting increased failure rates, complications, reoperations, operative time, and hospital length of stay for less experienced surgeons [48–50]. Interestingly, the learning curve for laparoscopic fundoplication is comparable to the West. In the era of minimal invasive surgery, laparoscopic techniques could be acquired without the prerequisite of open experience. Furthermore, under the laparoscopic view, the individual's anatomy is magnified, and details are more clearly demonstrated than in the open approach. In our center, the mean operative time for the first 10 LNF was 150 min, with gradual improvement to 90 min after 50 procedures. Over the past 20 years, the experience of LNF is getting mature rapidly within the Asia-Pacific region, and there is a trend toward laparoscopic partial fundoplication [51]. According to the international guidelines, it is recommended that young upper gastrointestinal surgeons have proctorship during their first 15–20 laparoscopic fundoplications [49].

Conclusion

It is now recognized that GERD is an emerging disease entity in Asia. It is foreseeable that the number of patients suffering from the disease will continue to increase in the Asia-Pacific region, and this poses a significant burden to the healthcare system. The particular diagnostic challenges could be overcome by means of improving awareness of the disease. It might be prudent to have regional validation for the use of the DeMeester score and symptom index, as the disease severity tends to be less with nonerosive GERD, yet patients' QOL are affected.

The majority of GERD patients are relatively young, and long-term acid suppressive therapy is usually required for symptomatic control. With the advancement in laparoscopic surgery, anti-reflux procedures become less invasive, with low perioperative morbidity and without mortality. Laparoscopic fundoplication, either complete or partial wrap, has become the alternative gold-standard treatment to medical therapy. More and more Asian gastrointestinal surgeons are competent in ARS, leading to an increasing tendency to offer this to patients, with higher acceptance. Although Asian countries have limited experience when compared to the Western countries, the overall surgical results from the East are encouraging. Training opportunities of the young surgeons are of paramount importance to meet the increasing need. Asia-Pacific consensus and recommendations concerning the surgical management of reflux disease are warranted to improve the overall surgical outcomes and patients' quality of life in the long run.

References

 1. Vakil N, van Zanten SV, Kahrilas P, Dent J, Joines R. Global consensus group. The Montreal definition and classification of gastroesophageal reflux disease: a global evidence-based consensus. Am J Gastroenterol. 2006;101(8):1900–20.
 2. Kahrilas PJ, Shaheen NJ, Vaezi MT, Hiltz SW, Black E, Modlin IM, et al. American Gastroenterological Association medical position statement on the management of gastroesophageal reflux disease. Gastroenterology. 2008;135(4):1383–91.
 3. Estscher GJ, REdmont EJ, Vititi LMH. Pathophysiology of gastroesophageal reflux disease. In: Hinder RA, editor. Gastroesophageal reflux disease. Austin TX: RG Landes; 1993. p. 7–29.
 4. Nebel OT, Fornes MT, Castell DO. Symptomatic gastroesophageal reflux: incidence and precipitating factors. Am J Dig Dis. 1976;21:953–6.
 5. El-Serag HB, Sweet S, Winchester CC, Dent J. Update on the epidemiology of gastroesophageal reflux disease: a systematic review. Gut. Jun 2014;63(6):871–80.
 6. Ehsani MJ, Maleki I, Mohammadzadeh F, Mashayekh A. Epidemiology of gastroesophageal reflux disease in Tehran. Trans J Gastroenterol Hepatol. 2007;22:1419–22.
 7. Bor S, Mandiracioglu A, Kitapcioglu G, Caymaz-Bor C, Gilber FJ. Gastroesophageal reflux disease in a low-income region in Turkey. Am J Gastroenterol. 2005;100:747–53.
 8. Dent J, El-Serag HB, Wallander MA, Johansson S. Epidemiology of gastro-oesophageal reflux disease: a systematic review. Gut. 2005;54:710–7.
 9. Lim SL, Goh WT, Lee JM, Ng TP, Ho KY. Changing prevalence of gastroesophageal reflux with changing time: longitudinal study in an Asian population. J Gastroenterol Hepatol. 2005;20:995–1001.
10. Manabe N, Haruma K, Mihara M, et al. The increasing incidence of reflux esophagitis during the past 20 years in Japan. Gastroenterology. 1999;116:A224.
11. Jung HK. Epidemiology of gastroesophageal reflux disease in Asia: a systemic review. J Neurogastroenterol Motil. 2011;17(1):14–27.
12. Du J, Liu J, Zhang H, Yu CH, Li YM. Risk factors for gastroesophageal reflux disease, reflux esophagitis an non-erosive reflux disease among Chinese patients undergoing upper gastrointestinal endoscopic examination. World J Gastroenterol. 2007;13:6009–15.
13. Ho YK, Cheung TK, Wong BC. Gastroesophageal reflux disease in Asian countries: disorder of nature or nurture? J Gastroenterol Hepatol. 2006;21(9):1362–5.
14. Fock KM, Talley NJ, Hunt RH, Fass R, Nandurkar S, Lam SK, et al. Report of the Asia Pacific consensus on the management of gastroesophageal reflux disease. J Gastroenterol Hepatol. 2004;19(4):357–67.
15. Fock KM, Talley NJ, Fass R, Goh KL, Katelaris P, Hunt R, et al. Asia- Pacific consensus on the management of gastroesophageal reflux disease: update. J Gastroenterol Hepatol. 2008;23(1):8–22.
16. Spechler SJ, Jain SK, Tendler DA, Parker RA. Racial differences in the frequency of symptoms and complications of gastro-oesophageal reflux disease. Aliment Pharmacol Ther. 2002;16(10):1795–800.
17. Ho KY, Ng WL, Kang JY, Yeoh KG. Gastroesophageal reflux disease is a common cause of noncardiac chest pain in a country with a low prevalence of reflux esophagitis. Dig Dis Sci. 1998;43(9):1991–7.
18. Wong WH, Lai KC, Lam KF, Hui WM, Hu WH, Lam CL, et al. Prevalence, clinical spectrum and health care utilization of gastro-oesophageal reflux disease in a Chinese population: a population-based study. Aliment Pharmacol Ther. 2003;18(6):595–604.

19. Wu JC. Gastroesophageal reflux disease: an Asian perspective. J Gastroenterol Hepatol. 2008;23:1785–93.
20. Johnson LF, DeMeester TR. Twenty-four-hour pH monitoring of the distal oesophagus. A quantitative measure of gastroesophageal reflux. Am J Gastroenterol. 1974;62(4):325–32.
21. Kahrilas PJ, Quigley EM. Clinical esophageal pH recording: a technical review for practical guideline development. Gastroenterology. 1996;110:1982–96.
22. Quigley EM. 24-h pH monitoring for gastroesophageal reflux disease: already standard but not yet gold? Am J Gastroenterol. 1992;87:1071–5.
23. Fass R, Naliboff B, Higa L, Johnson C, Kodner A, Munakata J, et al. Differential effect of long-term esophageal acid exposure on mechanosensitivity and chemosensitivity in humans. Gastroenterology. 1998;115(6):1363–73.
24. Kang JY, Tay HH, Yap I, Guan R, Lim KP, Math MV. Low frequency of endoscopic esophagitis in Asian patients. J Clin Gastroenterol. 1993;16:70–3.
25. Wong WM, Lam SK, Hui WM, Lai KC, Chan CK, Hu WH, et al. Long-term prospective follow-up of endoscopic oesophagitis in southern Chinese-prevalence and spectrum of the disease. Aliment Pharmacol Ther. 2002;16(12):2037–42.
26. Amano Y, Ishimura N, Furuta K, Akahashi Y, Chinuki D, Mishima Y, et al. Which landmark results in a more consistent diagnosis of Barrett's esophagus, the gastric folds or the palisade vessels? Gastrointest Endosc. 2006;64(2):206–11.
27. Kim JH, Rhee PL, Lee JH, Lee H, Choi YS, Son HJ, et al. Prevalence and risk factors of Barrett's esophagus in Korea. J Gastroenterol Hepatol. 2007;22(6):908–12.
28. Tseng PH, Lee YC, Chiu HM, Huang SP, Liao WC, Chen CC, et al. Prevalence and clinical characteristics of Barrett's esophagus in a Chinese general population. J Clin Gastroenterol. 2008;42(10):1074–9.
29. Wu JC, Chan FK, Ching JY, Leung WK, Lee YT, Sung JJ. Empirical treatment based on "typical" reflux symptoms is inappropriate in a population with a high prevalence of Helicobacter pylori infection. Gastrointest Endosc. 2002;55:461–5.
30. Ho KY, Gwee KA, Khor CH, Selamat DS, Wai CT, Yeoh KG. Empirical treatment for the management of patients presenting with uninvestigated reflux symptoms: a prospective study in an Asian primary care population. Aliment Pharmacol Ther. 2005;21:1313–20.
31. Wong WM, Lai KC, Hui WM, Lam KF, Huang JQ, Hu WH, et al. Double-blind, randomized controlled study to assess the effects of lansoprazole 30 mg and lansoprazole 15 mg on 24-h oesophageal and intragastric pH in Chinese subjects with gastro-oesophageal reflux disease. Aliment Pharmacol Ther. 2004;19(4):455–62.
32. Wu JC, Ching JYL, Au WL, et al. Clinical course of patients with non-erosive gastroesophageal reflux disease (NERD) on step-down acid suppressive therapy: a prospective cohort study. Gastroenterology. 2007;132(Suppl. 2):A139.
33. Lam SK. Differences in peptic ulcer between east and west. Baillieres Best Pract Res Clin Gastroenterol. 2000;14(1):41–52.
34. Ireland AC, Holloway RH, Toouli J, Dent J. Mechanisms underlying the antireflux action of fundoplication. Gut. 1993;34(3):303–8.
35. Johnson DA. Safety of proton pump inhibitors: current evidence for osteoporosis and interaction with antiplatelet agent. Curr Gastroenterol Rep. 2010;12:167–74.
36. Stefanidis D, Hope WW, Kohn GP, Reardon PR, Richardson WS, Fanelli RD. The SAGES guidelines committee. Guidelines for surgical treatment of gastroesophageal reflux disease. Surg Endosc. 2010;24:2647–69.
37. Nissen R. A simple operation for control of reflux esophagitis. Schweizersche Medizinische Wochenschrift. 1956;86(Suppl 20):590–2. German
38. Dallemagne B, Weerts JM, Jehaes C, Markiewicz S, Lombard R. Laparoscopic Nissen fundoplication: preliminary report. Surg Laparosc Endosc. 1991;1(3):138–43.
39. Kim KC, Park HJ, Yoon DS, Chi HS, Lee WH, Lee KS, et al. A case of paraesophageal hernia repaired by laparoscopic approach. Yonsei Med J. 1996;37:151–7.
40. Lee SK, Kim EK. Laparoscopic Nissen fundoplication in Korean patients with gastroesophageal reflux disease. Yonsei Med J. 2009;50(1):89–94.

41. Takeyama S, Numata A, Nenohi M, Shibata Y, Okushiba S, Katoh H. Laparoscopic Nissen fundoplication for gastroesophageal reflux disease in Japan. Surg Today. 2004;34(6):506–9.
42. Kumaresan S, Sudirman A, Ramesh G. Symptomatic outcome following laparoscopic anterior 180° partial fundoplication: our initial experience. Int Med Sci. 2010;4(2):128–32.
43. Catarci M, Gentileschi P, Papi C, Carrara A, Marrese R, Gaspari AL, et al. Evidence-based appraisal of antireflux fundoplication. Ann Surg. 2004;239:325–37.
44. Peters MJ, Mukhtar A, Yunus RM, Khan S, Pappalardo J, Memon B, et al. Meta-analysis of randomized clinical trials comparing open and laparoscopic anti-reflux surgery. Am J Gastroenterol. 2009;104:1548–61.
45. Cao Z, Cai W, Qin M, Zhao H, Yue P, Li Y. Randomized clinical trial of laparoscopic anterior 180° partial versus 360° Nissen fundoplication: 5-year results. Dis Esophagus. 2012;25:114–20.
46. Broeders JA, Roks DJ, Ahmed Ali U, Watson DI, Baigrie RJ, Cao Z, et al. Laparoscopic anterior 180-degree versus Nissen fundoplication for gastroesophageal reflux disease: systematic review and meta-analysis of randomized clinical trials. Ann Surg. 2013;257(5):850–9.
47. Neufeld M, Graham A. Levels of evidence available for techniques in antireflux surgery. Dis Esophagus. 2007;20:161–7.
48. Attwood SE, LUndell L, Ell C, Galmiche JP, Hatlebakk H, Fiocca R, et al. Standardization of surgical technique in antireflux surgery: the LOTUS trial experience. World J Surg. 2008;32(6):995–8.
49. Soper NJ, Dunnegan D. Anatomic fundoplication failure after laparoscopic antireflux surgery. Ann Surg. 1999;229(5):669–76.
50. Watson DI, Baigrie RJ, Jamieson GG. A learning curve for laparoscopic fundoplication. Definable, avoidable, or a waste of time? Ann Surg. 1996;224(2):198–203.
51. Deschamps C, Allen MS, Trastek VF, Johnson JO, Pairolero PC. Early experience and learning curve associated with laparoscopic Nissen fundoplication. J Thorac Cardiovasc Surg. 1998;115(2):281–4.

Barrett's Esophagus in the Asian Population

10

Khek Yu Ho

Abstract

In Asia, the prevalence of Barrett's esophagus derived from study of subjects undergoing endoscopy investigation is low compared to rates reported in Europe and North America. In Southeast and East Asia, where most of the existing data in Asia has been gathered, the prevalence of Barrett's esophagus in various populations studied mostly remains below 5%. As detection and, thereafter, diagnosis of Barrett's esophagus are highly dependent on recognition of the condition, there is evidence that lack of awareness of the condition in the region could have resulted in underdiagnosis of the disease. Despite this, the prevalence of Barrett's esophagus is beginning to rise in some parts of Asia.

Asians share many risk factors for Barrett's esophagus that are common with the populations in Europe and North America. Advancing age, male gender, and presence of reflux symptoms, esophagitis, or hiatal hernia have been identified as risk factors in Asians. Barrett's esophagus in Asians is characteristically milder than that of the Westerners, with nearly half of those affected being asymptomatic. Given that more than 90% of Barrett's esophagus cases in the Asian population are short-segment types, it is not surprising the incidence of Barrett's esophagus-associated esophageal adenocarcinoma is low in Asia. Endoscopic surveillance with random four-quadrant biopsies for patients with non-dysplastic Barrett's esophagus is not commonly carried out in Asian populations. Development of real-time in vivo and objective imaging technologies may help

K.Y. Ho (✉)
National University of Singapore/National University Hospital,
1E Kent Ridge Road NUHS Tower Block, Level 10, Singapore 119228, Singapore
e-mail: khek_yu_ho@nuhs.edu.sg

© Springer India 2018
P. Sharma et al. (eds.), *The Rise of Acid Reflux in Asia*,
DOI 10.1007/978-81-322-0846-4_10

123

overcome this limitation. Similar to the situation in the West, there is still no agreement on management strategies for Barrett's esophagus and its related neoplasia in Asia.

Keywords
Barrett's esophagus • Intestinal metaplasia • Asia • Population

Introduction

Barrett's adenocarcinoma is a rapidly rising malignancy in the West, and this trend has often been cited as the reason for recommending regular surveillance endoscopy in patients with Barrett's esophagus. On the other hand, Barrett's esophagus is often considered to be an uncommon upper gastrointestinal finding in the East. Where data are available, the prevalence of Barrett's esophagus is low in most parts of Asia. However, recent data indicating a slow-rising trend of Barrett's adenocarcinoma in Singapore [1] has prompted us to question whether the low prevalence of Barrett's esophagus in Asia is apparent rather than real and is due to the lack of awareness of this condition and, hence, its under-detection in the East. In the following sections, we will summarize the available data on the prevalence of Barrett's esophagus in Asian populations and show evidence suggesting a rising prevalence of Barrett's esophagus in Asia, we will examine the current endoscopic recognition and diagnosis of Barrett's esophagus as practiced in the Asian region and highlight the possibility of the condition being under-recognized and underdiagnosed in Asia, and we will discuss the genetic predispositions as well as other risk factors that have been observed in the various populations across Asia. We will also briefly introduce new technologies—including Raman spectroscopy and biomarker-based technology—that may enhance diagnosis of Barrett's esophagus given the challenges of recognizing and diagnosing this condition in Asia. Lastly, we will show that there is no uniform agreement on surveillance and treatment strategies for Barrett's esophagus and its related neoplasia in many centers in Asia.

Prevalence of Barrett's Esophagus in Asia

The epidemiology and etiology of Barrett's esophagus have been most extensively studied in Southeast and East Asia [2–5]. In these populations, the prevalence of Barrett's esophagus, based on histopathologic identification of intestinal metaplasia in endoscopically suspected Barrett's mucosa, ranged from 0.1 to 19.9%. However, excluding an exceptionally high rate reported in Japan by Amano et al. [6] where an astounding 19.9% of patients screened were found to have histologically confirmed Barrett's esophagus, the prevalence of Barrett's Esophagus in Southeast and East Asia lies within a low range of 0.1–5% [7–27].

In Japan, two large prospective multicenter studies, the Sendai Barrett's Esophagus Study (S-BEST) and the Far East Study (FEST) investigating the epidemiology of Barrett's esophagus on patients undergoing upper endoscopy during the period 1999 to 2000, found a 0.4–1.2% prevalence of Barrett's esophagus in the Japanese population [8]. The prevalence rates in the two studies were calculated based on a columnar-lined esophagus of any length with histological identification of specialized intestinal metaplasia. This is in contrast to the exceptionally high 19.9% prevalence rate of Barrett's esophagus (short segment in almost all cases) reported by Amano et al. in their study of 1668 subjects undergoing upper endoscopy in Japan during the period 2003–2004 [6]. It serves to note, though, in the latter study, only 31.8% of the Barrett's esophagus cases were of the intestinal-predominant mucin phenotype, while the rest, 68.2%, were of the gastric-predominant mucin phenotype. In a recent review by Manabe et al., involving 88,199 cases of upper endoscopy performed between 2008 and 2010 at 13 centers in Japan, the investigators identified long-segment Barrett's esophagus defined as a columnar-lined esophagus of more than 3 cm in length in only 13 (0.02%) of the subjects screened [9].

In a huge study covering 19,812 subjects in the Taiwan Chinese population who were undergoing health screening during the period 2003–2006, Tseng et al. reported a 0.1% prevalence of histologically confirmed Barrett's esophagus [10]. The majority of these patients (91.7%) had short-segment-type Barrett's esophagus. In another study published a year later, Chang et al. found a slightly higher (0.8%) prevalence of Barrett's esophagus, but then, of the 4797 subjects enrolled in this study, 3386 subjects were referral patients who were more likely to be symptomatic [11]. As expected, they found more histologically confirmed Barrett's esophagus cases among referral patients than among those undergoing health screening (1.1% in referral patients vs. 0.4% in those undergoing health screening). In another Taiwanese study by Kuo et al. which involved a population of 736 consecutive self-referred patients undergoing endoscopy for a variety of gastrointestinal symptoms in 2007 [12], they found a higher prevalence of Barrett's esophagus (3.8%) in patients with gastroesophageal reflux disease compared with the total study population (1.8%).

A nationwide study conducted in Korea by Park et al. found a Barrett's esophagus prevalence of 0.8% among 25,536 subjects who underwent upper endoscopy screening during the period [13]. In a study conducted at 11 Korean tertiary referral centers which evaluated 2048 patients undergoing endoscopy in 2006, Lee et al. reported a Barrett's esophagus prevalence of 1.0% [14]. In a more recent study by Choi et al. on 4002 patients who underwent upper endoscopy in 2012, a similar proportion (1.0%) of patients were found to have histologically proven specialized intestinal metaplasia in the distal esophagus [15].

In one of the largest studies, involving 139,416 patients undergoing screening endoscopy in Eastern China which spanned over a 7-year period from 2005 to 2012, Zhang et al. found a 0.2% prevalence of histologically confirmed Barrett's esophagus [16]. As with other Asian populations, most cases diagnosed (>90%) were short-segment Barrett's esophagus. Two other studies by Peng et al. and Xiong et al. reported prevalence of 0.5% and 1.0% in a health screening population of 2580 individuals without reflux symptoms and a cohort of 2580 patients who were investigated for upper gastrointestinal symptoms, respectively [17, 18]. However, higher prevalence was reported in two recent studies which evaluated only symptomatic patients. A study by Zhang et al. in a central China population (Luoyang city) found a 4.6% prevalence of Barrett's esophagus among 593 consecutive patients presenting with upper gastrointestinal symptoms [19]. In another study conducted in 2009 in Northwest China, Barrett's esophagus was diagnosed in 6.1% of 528 patients with gastroesophageal reflux disease [20]. In both studies, the subjects enrolled were patients undergoing endoscopy for investigation of upper gastrointestinal symptoms or already had gastroesophageal reflux disease.

In Malaysia, reported prevalence of Barrett's esophagus among patients who underwent endoscopy for investigation of upper gastrointestinal symptoms ranged from 0.8 to 6% [21–23]. Limited data from Singapore and the Philippines showed equally low prevalence of Barrett's esophagus [3, 23–28].

Data from most parts of India have reported a slightly higher prevalence of histologically confirmed Barrett's esophagus. Dhawan et al. reported 6% of 271 patients undergoing diagnostic upper gastrointestinal endoscopy had specialized columnar epithelium, while Mathew et al. reported 9% of the 278 patients with gastroesophageal reflux disease they studied had specialized intestinal metaplasia [4, 25]. These prevalence rates are closer to that reported among Indian diasporas elsewhere [26].

Is Barrett's Esophagus an Under-Recognized Disease in the East?

Awareness of the disease and diagnostic practices are known to influence the rate of diagnosis. Past reports of low incidence of Barrett's esophagus in Asia could, in part, be attributed to the lack of awareness and therefore underdiagnosis of the disease. In Singapore, we conducted a retrospective study on 29,447 esophagogastro-duodenoscopy procedures performed from the year 2006 to 2010, a period which witnessed increasing awareness of Barrett's esophagus in our hospital. The incidence of histologically confirmed Barrett's esophagus increased from a low rate of <0.1% in the year 2006 to >0.2% in the years 2008, 2009, and 2010 [3]. We found no significant difference in the Barrett's esophagus versus non-Barrett's esophagus patient cohorts over the years, whether it is in terms of race, gender, or age. The increase in the incidence of Barrett's esophagus in the latter years was most likely a result of more diagnoses made as awareness of the disease condition increased and doctors gained more experiences in the endoscopic investigation of the disease. Indeed, a recent study conducted in Singapore found that formal training in the use of the Prague C and M criteria for the endoscopic recognition and grading of Barrett's esophagus facilitated endoscopists' detection of the disease and led to significantly higher diagnostic yield during endoscopy [27].

Another major cause of concern in Asia is that different diagnostic criteria and investigation methods are used in different countries, thus making head-to-head comparison of diagnostic data collected across geographical borders inappropriate. Unlike in Europe and North America, there is a lack of consistency in the diagnostic criteria and methods used in the investigation of Barrett's esophagus in Asia. In particular, there are different endoscopic criteria for defining Barrett's esophagus. The term "Barrett's esophagus" is often used interchangeably with "columnar-lined esophagus." The different definitions of the gastroesophageal junction might, to a certain extent, account for discrepancy in reported prevalence of Barrett's esophagus across Asia. Currently, diagnosis of Barrett's esophagus in Asian populations is mainly based on the presence of columnar-type epithelium at endoscopy, with histopathologic finding of intestinal metaplasia, but depending on criteria used by the investigator, the presence of intestinal metaplasia might not be necessary for a diagnosis of Barrett's esophagus [28, 29]. In Japan, the investigation and diagnosis criteria for Barrett's esophagus differ substantially from the rest of Asia and the world [30]. Unlike in other East Asian countries, the presence of specialized columnar metaplasia is not considered to be important for diagnosis of Barrett's esophagus in Japan. Besides, while most countries in Asia use the proximal margin of the gastric folds as the gastroesophageal junction, in Japan and Korea, the distal limit of the lower esophageal palisade vessels is usually regarded as the gastroesophageal junction, and the designated area of the columnar-lined esophagus is anatomically defined by the distal limit of the lower esophageal palisade vessels [31].

In contrast to studies from Western countries, most cases of Barrett's esophagus found in Asian populations are short segments. This contributes to the third challenge in the investigation of Barrett's esophagus in Asia. As we know, endoscopic diagnosis of short-segment-type Barrett's esophagus, particularly those <1 cm, has been found to be difficult and highly unreliable. In a recent multicenter study conducted by the Asian Barrett's Consortium, it was found that the interobserver reliability for the endoscopic diagnosis of Barrett's esophagus, expressed as intraclass correlation coefficients, was extremely low, at 0.18 and 0.21 for C and M values, respectively. This was deemed unacceptable [32]. Besides, the use of four-quadrant biopsy protocol is not a standard practice in many Asian countries. A study conducted in Taiwan revealed possible underestimation of the true prevalence when four-quadrant biopsy protocol is not used [11]. Using standardized four-quadrant biopsy protocol, the investigators found endoscopically suspected Barrett's esophagus and histologically proven Barrett's esophagus in 1.9 and 0.9% of the study population, respectively. Whereas, on the basis of at least two biopsies, the same investigators found in a retrospective study prevalence of only 0.3 and 0.1% endoscopically suspected Barrett's esophagus and histologically proven Barrett's esophagus, respectively [10].

Can Advanced Imaging Technologies and Biomarkers Improve Diagnosis of Barrett's Esophagus, Especially in the East?

While imaging technologies capable of providing significant enhancement to endoscopic evaluations of disease are available, these technologies rely heavily on the operator's ability to interpret the images. To overcome the issue of learning curve and dependency on the operator's subjectivity in interpretation of endoscopic findings, Raman spectroscopy is now being evaluated at our center. Data derived from a study on patients with Barrett's esophagus show there is immense potential for the system to be applied for real-time in vivo diagnosis of Barrett's esophagus and its associated esophageal neoplasia [33]. This technology has several advantages: (1) the probe can be inserted via the working channel of the endoscopy to be placed focally at the lesion, (2) the diagnosis can be displayed real time on a monitor, and (3) no contrast is required for the generation of the spectroscopic images.

The second strategy to aid diagnosis of Barrett's esophagus is the use of bio-markers. By mining expression data sets of the Barrett's stem cell clones, our team is working on identifying unique cell surface markers of the Barrett's stem cells against which antibodies or aptamers can be developed and used to aid the endoscopist in identifying regions of atypia for biopsy, perform real-time diagnosis, and stratify patients during the examination [34, 35].

Is Barrett's Esophagus Rising in Prevalence in the East?

There is some evidence that the prevalence of Barrett's esophagus may be increasing in Asia. Comparing a study done on 4002 patients who underwent endoscopy in 2012 [14] with an earlier study conducted on 70,103 subjects undergoing their first upper endoscopies during the period from 1997 to 2004 in Korea, Choi et al. reported the prevalence of Barrett's esophagus as defined by histologically identifiable specialized intestinal metaplasia in columnar-lined esophagus appeared to have risen over the decade [16]. In the Philippines, among 15,981 patients diagnosed with erosive esophagitis from 1994 to 1997 and from 2000 to 2003, endoscopically visible Barrett's segment was found in 3.2% of the patients in the earlier period and 5% of the patients in the later period [36]. However, it should be understood that diagnosing BE in patients with erosive esophagitis is very challenging and predicting the true incidence of BE using these populations may be difficult. As mentioned previously, a retrospective review of 29,447 esophagogastroduodenoscopy procedures carried out at the National University Hospital, Singapore, during the period 2006 to 2010 revealed that incidence of histologically confirmed Barrett's esophagus in the mixed population undergoing endoscopy for a variety of indications had increased from a low rate of <0.1% in the year 2006 to >0.2% in the years 2008, 2009, as well as 2010 [3].

Barrett's Esophagus Is Mostly Short Segment in Asian Populations

As alluded to previously, Barrett's esophagus seen in the populations of Southeast and East Asia are shorter in length as compared to that found in their Caucasian counterparts in Europe and America. Reports from across Asia show that 90–97% of Barrett's esophagus cases seen in this part of the world are short-segment-type Barrett's esophagus and many of them are ultrashort-segment Barrett's esophagus of <1 cm in length [6, 9, 10, 14, 16, 37]. In a study done in China, investigators found that island-type Barrett's esophagus was predominant (57%), with 37% of the cases being Barrett's esophagus with special intestinal metaplasia [38].

Risk Factors for Barrett's Esophagus

Genetic Predisposition to Barrett's Esophagus

The fact that Caucasians are more prone than Asians to develop long-segment Barrett's esophagus and associated adenocarcinoma is now common knowledge [39, 40]. There is credible evidence of ethnic disparity in predisposition to Barrett's esophagus in certain parts of Asia and among specific racial ethnic groups. Rajendra et al. first reported that among the three major ethnic groups (Indians, Malays, and Chinese) in Southeast Asia, the Indians had the highest prevalence of Barrett's esophagus when compared with the Chinese ($P < 0.05$) and the Malays ($P < 0.01$) [23]. In a follow-up study a few years later, Rajendra et al. further confirmed that being Indian is a risk factor for Barrett' esophagus [41]. They deduced that the risk may be related to the Caucasian genetic makeup of Indians and inferred that the HLA-B07 gene commonly found in Indian (South Asian) and Caucasian populations, but not in Orientals, may confer an increased risk for Barrett's esophagus [43].

Advancing Age Is a Common Risk Factor

Association of advancing age with Barrett's esophagus has been reported by almost all risk studies conducted in various populations across Asia. By the time of first diagnosis, Asian Barrett's esophagus patients would usually be in their fifth or sixth decade of life. In one of the recent reviews of population-based studies of Barrett's esophagus conducted in ethnic Chinese populations in Taiwan, mainland China, and Hong Kong SAR, advancing age was found to be a prominent independent risk factor for Barrett's esophagus in the Asian populations studied [5]. Increasing prevalence of Barrett's esophagus with advancing age is also clearly shown in one of the largest study involving 139,416 subjects conducted over a 7-year period in Eastern China ($x^2 = 9.25$, $p < 0.0001$) [16]. In a study on a population of 4002 Koreans undergoing endoscopy, the investigators found that the mean age of subjects with Barrett's esophagus was significantly higher than of those without Barrett's esophagus [14]. Likewise, in Japan, in a population of 869 Japanese subjects undergoing health checks, the individual's age was found to be significantly associated with the prevalence of Barrett's epithelium [44].

Despite Barrett's esophagus being associated with advancing age, it has been noted that some Asian Barrett's esophagus patients may be susceptible to Barrett's esophagus at an earlier age than their Western counterparts. In a review of 308 papers reporting studies conducted on various populations in China and involving a total of 4120 subjects undergoing endoscopy for various upper gastrointestinal symptoms, investigators found that the average age of Barrett's esophagus diagnosis in Chinese was 53.2 years, which is several years younger than the reported average age in European populations [38]. Risk at an even younger age has been noted in populations studied in India. Investigators there showed that age $\geq$ 45 years is a risk factor for specialized intestinal metaplasia in the Indian population studied [25]. The reason for the lower age of diagnosis of Barrett's esophagus in some Asians is unclear.

Gender: More Males than Females Develop Barrett's Esophagus

A preponderance of males among Asian patients with Barrett's esophagus has been reported by a few investigators. In a cohort of 4120 patients undergoing endoscopy for various upper gastrointestinal symptoms in China, investigators found a male/female ratio of 2:1 in those diagnosed with Barrett's esophagus, which is close to the 2:1 ratio reported in Europeans [38]. In Korea, a recent study showed a significantly higher proportion of males in subjects with Barrett's esophagus than in the rest of study population who do not have Barrett's esophagus [14]. However, other studies—including a study by Kuo et al. in Taiwan, Lee et al. in Korea, Zhang et al. in China, and Mathew et al. in India—found no gender difference in the risk for Barrett's esophagus [12, 14, 16, 25].

Gastroesophageal Reflux Disease and Reflux Esophagitis Are Primary Risk Factors

Almost in all populations studied across Asia, investigators have found varying degrees of association between reflux symptoms and Barrett's esophagus. In addition, erosive esophagitis has also been found to increase the odds for development of Barrett's esophagus. In the Japanese population, Akiyama et al. showed, using a multivariate model, severe erosive esophagitis was significantly associated with the prevalence of Barrett's epithelium (OR = 5.2; 95% CI, 3.4–7.7), as well as with its progression [43]. In Korea, similar findings were found in a study of 2048 endoscopy patients, in which those with reflux esophagitis were found to be having the highest odds for developing Barrett's esophagus (OR 10.3) [13]. A similar risk for Barrett's esophagus in presence of reflux esophagitis (OR 4.4; 95% CI, 1.22–16.17) was reported in a study involving 2022 patients in Southeastern China [17]. Longer duration of gastroesophageal reflux disease was also found to be a risk factor for the development of Barrett's esophagus. Among 736 consecutive Chinese patients undergoing upper endoscopy for a variety of gastrointestinal symptoms in Taiwan, the duration of gastroesophageal reflux disease was found an independent risk factor for Barrett's esophagus (OR = 4.2; 95% CI, 1.2–4.8; P = 0.03) [12].

There is an apparent lack of association between gastroesophageal reflux disease and short-segment Barrett's esophagus in Asian populations. In fact, nearly half of the Asian patients with Barrett's esophagus do not have a history of gastroesophageal reflux disease, and this is believed to be related to the dominance of short-segment Barrett's esophagus in Asians [1–5, 44]. In a study conducted on a huge ethnic Chinese population by Zhang et al., about half of the patients diagnosed with Barrett's esophagus exhibited no reflux symptoms; only 7.3% of Barrett's esophagus patients diagnosed satisfied the diagnostic criteria of gastroesophageal reflux disease based on their GERDQ symptom scores [16]. Similarly, a 2011 literature review of studies on gastroesophageal reflux disease in Asia found only 60.1% of subjects with Barrett's esophagus having reflux symptoms [4]. In Korea, a large nationwide study conducted in 2009 found 39.9% of Barrett's esophagus patients had no reflux symptoms and 77.7% did not have endoscopic erosions [15]. The lack of evidence directly associating gastroesophageal reflux disease with short-segment Barrett's esophagus concurs with findings from international data showing that although reflux symptoms increase the odds of having long-segment Barrett's esophagus, the symptoms are not associated with short-segment Barrett's esophagus [45].

Hiatal Hernia: Another Major Risk Factor

A review of population-based studies conducted in ethnic Chinese populations in Taiwan, mainland China, and Hong Kong SAR showed hiatal hernia as one of two most prominent independent risk factors for Barrett's esophagus [5]. Among the studies reviewed was one study of a population of 736 consecutive Taiwanese patients undergoing diagnostic endoscopy for a variety of gastrointestinal symptoms that determined that hiatal hernia was the strongest among a few independent risk factors evaluated for the development of Barrett's esophagus (OR = 4.7; 95% CI, 1.3–17.7; P = 0.02) [12]. In Korea, a study on 215 Barrett's esophagus patients revealed that hiatal hernia was the strongest risk factor for Barrett's esophagus [15]. This observation was echoed in a later study of 2048 patients undergoing endoscopy in a Korean hospital, which reported presence of hiatal hernia as a significant risk factor for Barrett's esophagus (OR 5.1; 95% CI, 3.05–8.21) [13]. In Japan, hiatal hernia was associated both with Barrett's esophagus and the length of Barrett's esophagus, and it was also found to be an independent predictor of circumferential-type short-segment Barrett's esophagus (OR 4.5; 95% CI, 3.23–5.45) [37]. In Malaysia, hiatus hernia was found positively associated with Barrett's metaplasia (OR, 5.4; 95% CI, 3.41–8.57) [23]. Significant association between hiatal hernia and columnar-lined esophagus was also reported by Navarathne et al. in their study of 1150 South Asian patients who underwent endoscopy for various indications [46].

Little Evidence of Obesity as a Risk for Barrett's Esophagus

Few studies in Asia actually confirmed obesity as a risk factor for Barrett's esophagus. A large study by Fujimoto et al. on a population of 42,862 Japanese adults showed body mass index (BMI) > 25 kg/m^2 was not associated with Barrett's esophagus [47]. In Korea, similar observations have been reported. In a large retrospective analysis of 70,103 subjects who underwent upper endoscopy, the investigators found no relationship between BMI > 25 kg/m^2 and Barrett's esophagus [48]. Similarly, in South Asia, BMI >30 kg/m^2 was found not to predispose the subject to Barrett's esophagus in a study by Bamanikar et al. [49]. Thus, at present, there is insufficient evidence in the studied Asian populations to prove that obesity per se predisposes an individual to Barrett's esophagus.

Controversial Effects of Tobacco and Alcohol Consumption

The impact of tobacco and alcohol consumption on the development of Barrett's esophagus is uncertain in Asia. In a study on Japanese patients, Akiyama et al. found that a smoking habit was significantly associated with increased prevalence of Barrett's epithelium (OR = 1.9), but drinking alcohol was not associated [43]. In Taiwan, a study on 19,812 subjects reported that smoking and alcohol might be associated with the presence of Barrett's esophagus [10]. But among Indian subjects, consumption of tobacco or alcohol was found to not be associated with Barrett's esophagus [25].

Impact of *Helicobacter pylori* Infection

A recent meta-analysis of 49 studies worldwide suggests that *Helicobacter pylori* infection is associated with a reduced risk of Barrett's esophagus [50]. In Japan, two studies by Abe et al. (in 2009 and 2011) found that *H. pylori* was inversely associated with the development of Barrett's esophagus [51, 52]. The historical lower prevalence of gastroesophageal reflux disease and Barrett's esophagus in Asia had been attributed to the higher prevalence of *H. pylori* in the region, as compared to the West. The increasing prevalence of gastroesophageal reflux disease, the precursor of Barrett's esophagus, in the past decades is believed to be a result of declining *H. pylori* infection in the region. This supposition is supported by data in a number of studies conducted in Asia, including the study by Ho et al. and Rajendra et al. [53, 54].

Malignant Transformation of Barrett's Esophagus

In Asia, where the incidence of esophageal adenocarcinoma is extremely low, esophageal adenocarcinoma associated with Barrett's esophagus is rarely seen. Despite the recent increase in prevalence of Barrett's esophagus in some parts of Asia, the incidence of esophageal adenocarcinoma has remained low in Asia as a whole. In East Asia, incidence of esophageal adenocarcinoma has been reported to be increasing in Japan and Singapore. In Japan, during the period from 1960 to

1995, the annual death rate from esophageal adenocarcinoma increased from 3.7 to 6.9 per 100,000 population [8]. In Singapore, age-standardized incidence rates for esophageal adenocarcinoma rose from 0 to 0.54 per 100,000 men and from 0.03 to 0.13 per 100,000 women between 1968 and 2002 [55]. Despite these increases in incidence, the absolute number of esophageal adenocarcinoma cases seen today remains very low in these countries, as compared to that seen in the West. Contrasting the development in Singapore and Japan, the incidence of esophageal adenocarcinoma declined in Hong Kong and remained unchanged in Taiwan and Korea [56–58]. In Hong Kong, a study of 10,751 new cases of esophageal neoplasm during the period 1984 to 1988 showed that the relative ratio of esophageal adenocarcinoma versus esophageal squamous cell carcinoma decreased from 11.7% then to 6.4% during the period 1998 to 2003 [56]. In Korea, a retrospective review of 16,811 cases of esophageal squamous cell carcinoma or gastric noncardiac adenocarcinoma diagnosed between 1992 and 2006 discovered no increase in the ratio of incidence of adenocarcinoma to non-adenocarcinoma of the esophagogastric junction [57]. In Taiwan, although a significant increase in the incidence of esophageal squamous cell carcinoma was seen during the period 1979 to 2003, there was no change in the incidence of esophageal adenocarcinoma [58]. In China, despite a high incidence of esophageal squamous cell carcinoma in its population, the incidence of esophageal adenocarcinoma remains extremely low and accounted for only about 1% of all distal esophageal cancers diagnosed [5].

Management of Barrett's Esophagus and Its Associated Neoplasia in Asia

Endoscopic surveillance with random four-quadrant biopsies for patients with non-dysplastic Barrett's esophagus is deemed by many to be impractical to be carried out in Asian populations. Firstly, the incidence of esophageal adenocarcinoma is very low in Asia. In fact, the current recommended regimen for Barrett's esophagus surveillance has been called into question in the light of new findings showing the lack of justification for rigorous surveillance of non-dysplastic Barrett's esophagus. According to a recent population-based study involving 11,028 patients with Barrett's esophagus, the absolute annual risk of Barrett-related esophageal adenocarcinoma is only about 0.12% and well below the assumed 0.5% rate used in development of current surveillance guidelines [59]. The risk of esophageal adenocarcinoma is expected to be even lower in Asian populations, as the odds for short-segment Barrett's esophagus to develop into cancer are lower. Secondly, most Asian patients have short-segment Barrett's esophagus, in which case obtaining four-quadrant biopsies within the tiny Barrett's segment is practically near to impossible. Hence, it is unlikely that rigorous surveillance of non-dysplastic Barrett's esophagus would pick up in Asia any time soon.

Management for esophageal neoplasia has evolved in recent time due to advances in endoscopic techniques and ablative therapies. In a study of management strategies for Barrett's esophagus and its associated neoplasia in Korea, Singapore, and

Japan, the authors found several interesting observations. All of the Japanese endoscopists preferred endoscopic resection for Barrett's adenocarcinoma, whereas a quarter to approximately half of the Korean and Singaporean endoscopists preferred surgical resection. For Barrett's esophagus with low-grade dysplasia, treatment with a proton pump inhibitor was the preferred strategy in Japan, whereas in Korea and Singapore, endoscopic treatment was preferred [60].

Conclusion

The prevalence of Barrett's esophagus in most Asian populations studied is low compared to the rates reported in Western populations. The histological low prevalence rates reported in various parts of Asia could have been attributed, at least in part, to underdiagnosis and/or lack of awareness of the condition. There is evidence that the prevalence of Barrett's esophagus is rising in some parts of Asia. Most cases of Barrett's esophagus in Asia are short segment, and half of the cases are asymptomatic. Although patients with Barrett's esophagus in both Asia and the West appear to share similar risk factors such as male gender, older age, and longer duration of reflux symptoms, patients in some parts of Asia tend to be diagnosed with Barrett's esophagus at a younger age—at least 10 years earlier than when it occurs in Caucasians.

Esophageal adenocarcinoma is rare in Asia, and this may be due to the dominance of short-segment Barrett's esophagus in Asians. Endoscopic surveillance with random four-quadrant biopsies for patients with non-dysplastic Barrett's esophagus is not commonly carried out in Asian populations. Development of real-time in vivo and objective imaging technologies with optical biopsy capabilities may help overcome this limitation. There is still no agreement on management strategies for Barrett's esophagus and its related neoplasia in Asia. As the awareness of the disease continues to increase, we are likely to see more cases of Barrett's esophagus detected and diagnosed in Asia.

References

1. Ho KY. From GERD to Barrett's esophagus: is the pattern in Asia mirroring that in the west? J Gastroenterol Hepatol. 2011;26(5):816–24.
2. Hongo M, Nagasaki Y, Shoji T. Epidemiology of esophageal cancer: orient to occident. Effects of chronology, geography and ethnicity. J Gastroenterol Hepatol. 2009;24(5):729–35.
3. Ho KY. Asia-Pacific Barrett's consortium. Is Barrett's esophagus an over-hyped disease in the west, and an underdiagnosed disease in the East? Dig Endosc. 2013;25(Suppl 2):157–61.
4. Jung HK. Epidemiology of gastroesophageal reflux disease in Asia: a systematic review. J Neurogastroenterol Motil. 2011;17(1):14–27.
5. Huang Q, Fang DC, Yu CG, Zhang J, Chen MH. Barrett's esophagus-related diseases remain uncommon in China. J Dig Dis. 2011;12(6):420–7.
6. Amano Y, Kushiyama Y, Yuki T, Takahashi Y, Moriyama I, Fukuhara H, et al. Prevalence of and risk factors for Barrett's esophagus with intestinal predominant mucin phenotype. Scand J Gastroenterol. 2006;41(8):873–9.

7. Fock KM, Ang TL. Global epidemiology of Barrett's esophagus. Expert Rev Gastroenterol Hepatol. 2011 Feb;5(1):123–30.
8. Hongo M. Review article: Barrett's oesophagus and carcinoma in Japan. Aliment Pharmacol Ther. 2004 Dec;20(Suppl 8):50–4.
9. Manabe N, Matsueda K, Haruma K, Yamamoto H, Matsumoto H, et al. The incidence of Barrett's esophagus and adenocarcinoma are still low in Japan. Gastroenterology. 2011;140(5):S222.
10. Tseng PH, Lee YC, Chiu HM, Huang SP, Liao WC, Chen CC, et al. Prevalence and clinical characteristics of Barrett's esophagus in a Chinese general population. J Clin Gastroenterol. 2008;42(10):1074–9.
11. Chang CY, Lee YC, Lee CT, Tu CH, Hwang JC, Chiang H, et al. The application of Prague C and M criteria in the diagnosis of Barrett's esophagus in an ethnic Chinese population. Am J Gastroenterol. 2009;104(1):13–20.
12. Kuo CJ, Lin CH, Liu NJ, Wu RC, Tang JH, Cheng CL. Frequency and risk factors for Barrett's esophagus in Taiwanese patients: a prospective study in a tertiary referral center. Dig Dis Sci. 2010;55(5):1337–43.
13. Park JJ, Kim JW, Kim HJ, Chung MG, Park SM, Baik GH, et al. The prevalence of and risk factors for Barrett's esophagus in a Korean population: s nationwide multicenter prospective study. J Clin Gastroenterol. 2009;43(10):907–14.
14. Lee IS, Choi SC, Shim KN, Jee SR, Huh KC, Lee JH. Lee et al. prevalence of Barrett's esophagus remains low in the Korean population: nationwide cross-sectional prospective multicenter study. Dig Dis Sci. 2010;55(7):1932–9.
15. Choi CY, Suh S, Park JS, Lee HJ, Lee JS, Choi HS, et al. The prevalence of Barrett's esophagus and the comparison of Barrett's esophagus with cardiac intestinal metaplasia in the health screening at a secondary care hospital. Korean J Gastroenterol. 2012;60(4):219–23.
16. Zhang M, Fan XS, Zou XP. The prevalence of Barrett's esophagus remains low in eastern China. Single-center 7-year descriptive study. Saudi Med J. 2012;33(12):1324–9.
17. Xiong LS, Cui Y, Wang JP, Wang JH, Xue L, Hu PJ, et al. Prevalence and risk factors of Barrett's esophagus in patients undergoing endoscopy for upper gastrointestinal symptoms. J Dig Dis. 2010;11(2):83–7.
18. Peng S, Cui Y, Xiao YL, Xiong LS, Hu PJ, Li CJ, et al. Prevalence of erosive esophagitis and Barrett's esophagus in the adult Chinese population. Endoscopy. 2009;41(12):1011–7.
19. Zhang RG, Wang CS, Gao CF. Prevalence and pathogenesis of Barrett's esophagus in Luoyang. China Asian Pac J Cancer Prev. 2012;13(5):2185–91.
20. Yin C, Zhang J, Gao M, Shen Q, Dong L. Epidemiological investigation of Barrett's esophagus in patients with gastroesophageal reflux disease in Northwest China. J Med College PLA. 2012;27(4):187–97.
21. Lee YY, Tuan Sharif SE, Syed Abd Aziz SH, Raj SM. Barrett's esophagus in an area with an exceptionally low prevalence of helicobacter pylori Infection. ISRN Gastroenterol. 2011;2011:394734.
22. Rosaida MS, Goh KL. Gastro-oesophageal reflux disease, reflux oesophagitis and non-erosive reflux disease in a multiracial Asian population: a prospective, endoscopy based study. Eur J Gastroenterol Hepatol. 2004 May;16(5):495–501.
23. Rajendra S, Kutty K, Karim N. Ethnic differences in the prevalence of endoscopic esophagitis and Barrett's esophagus: the long and short of it all. Dig Dis Sci. 2004;49(2):237–42.
24. Dhawan PS, Alvares JF, Vora IM, Joseph TK, Bhatia SJ, Amarapurkar AD, et al. Prevalence of short segments of specialized columnar epithelium in distal esophagus: association with gastroesophageal reflux. Indian J Gastroenterol. 2001;20(4):144–7.
25. Mathew P, Joshi AS, Shukla A, Bhatia SJ. Risk factors for Barrett's esophagus in Indian patients with gastroesophageal reflux disease. J Gastroenterol Hepatol. 2011;26(7):1151–6.
26. Goh KL. Changing epidemiology of gastroesophageal reflux disease in the Asian-Pacific region: an overview. J Gastroenterol Hepatol. 2004;19(Suppl 3):S22–5.
27. Li XH, Chang CY, Goto H, et al. Formal training in the endoscopic recognition of Barrett's esophagus improves detection rate and increases diagnostic yield. J Gastroenterol Hepatol. 2011;26(Suppl 5):213.

28. Wang KK, Sampliner RE. Practice parameters Committee of the American College of gastro-enterology. Updated guidelines 2008 for the diagnosis, surveillance and therapy of Barrett's esophagus. Am J Gastroenterol. 2008 Mar;103(3):788–97.
29. Playford RJ. New British Society of Gastroenterology (BSG) guidelines for the diagnosis and management of Barrett's oesophagus. Gut. 2006;55(4):442.
30. Ishimura N, Amano Y, Appelman HD, Penagini R, Tenca A, Falk GW, et al. Barrett's esophagus: endoscopic diagnosis. Ann N Y Acad Sci. 2011;1232:53–75.
31. Ogiya K, Kawano T, Ito E, Nakajima Y, Kawada K, Nishikage T, et al. Lower esophageal palisade vessels and the definition of Barrett's esophagus. Dis Esophagus. 2008;21:645–9.
32. Lee YC, Cook MB, Bhatia S, Chow WH, El-Omar EM, Goto H, et al. Interobserver reliability in the endoscopic diagnosis and grading of Barrett's esophagus: an Asian multinational study. Endoscopy. 2010;42(9):699–704.
33. Bergholt MS, Zheng W, Ho KY, Teh M, Yeoh KG, So JB, et al. Fiberoptic confocal Raman spectroscopy for real-time in vivo diagnosis of dysplasia in Barrett's esophagus. Gastroenterology. 2014;146(1):27–32.
34. Wang X, Ouyang H, Yamamoto Y, Kumar PA, Wei TS, Dagher R, et al. Residual embryonic cells as precursors of a Barrett's-like metaplasia. Cell. 2011;145(7):1023–35.
35. Xian W, Ho KY, Crum CP, McKeon F. Cellular origin of Barrett's esophagus: controversy and therapeutic implications. Gastroenterology. 2012;142(7):1424–30.
36. Sollano JD, Wong SN, Andal-Gamutan T, Chan MM, Carpio RE, Tady CS, et al. Erosive esophagitis in the Philippines: a comparison between two time periods. J Gastroenterol Hepatol. 2007;22(10):1650–5.
37. Okita K, Amano Y, Takahashi Y, Mishima Y, Moriyama N, Ishimura N, et al. Barrett's esophagus in Japanese patients: its prevalence, form, and elongation. J Gastroenterol. 2008;43:928–34.
38. Chen X, Zhu LR, Hou XH. The characteristics of Barrett's esophagus: an analysis of 4120 cases in China. Dis Esophagus. 2009;22(4):348–53.
39. Kang JY. Systematic review: geographical and ethnic differences in gastro-oesophageal reflux disease. Aliment Pharmacol Ther. 2004;20(7):705–17.
40. Sharma P, Wani S, Romero Y, Johnson D, Hamilton F. Racial and geographic issues in gastroesophageal reflux disease. Am J Gastroenterol. 2008;103(11):2669–80.
41. Rajendra S. Barrett's oesophagus in Asians--are ethnic differences due to genes or the environment? J Intern Med. 2011;270(5):421–7.
42. Rajendra S, Ackroyd R, Murad S, Mohan C, Too CL, Azrena A. Barrett's oesophagus and HLA-B*0702/HLA-B*0706. Aliment Pharmacol Ther. 2006;23(9):1375–6.
43. Akiyama T, Inamori M, Akimoto K, Iida H, Mawatari H, Endo H, et al. Risk factors for the progression of endoscopic Barrett's epithelium in Japan: a multivariate analysis based on the Prague C & M Criteria. Dig Dis Sci. 2009;54:1702–7.
44. Chang CY, Cook MB, Lee YC, Lin JT, Ando T, Bhatia S, et al. Current status of Barrett's esophagus research in Asia. J Gastroenterol Hepatol. 2011;26(2):240–6.
45. Taylor JB, Rubenstein JH. Meta-analyses of the effect of symptoms of gastroesophageal reflux on the risk of Barrett's esophagus. Am J Gastroenterol. 2010;105(8):1729–37.
46. Navarathne NM, Abeysuriya V, Ileperuma A, Thoufeek UL. Endoscopic observations around the gastroesophageal junction in patients with symptomatic gastroesophageal reflux disease in South Asia. Indian J Gastroenterol. 2010;29(5):184–6.
47. Fujimoto A, Hoteya S, Iizuka T, Ogawa O, Mitani T, Kuroki Y, et al. Obesity and gastrointestinal diseases. Gastroenterol Res Pract. 2013;2013:760574.
48. Kim JH, Rhee PL, Lee JH, Lee H, Choi YS, Son HJ, et al. Prevalence and risk factors of Barrett's esophagus in Korea. J Gastroenterol Hepatol. 2007;22(6):908–12.
49. Bamanikar AA, Diwan AG, Benoj DE, Bamanikar SA. Barrett's metaplasia in Indian obese male patients with gastro-oesophageal reflux disease. J Indian Med Assoc. 2011;109(7):483–4.
50. Fischbach LA, Nordenstedt H, Kramer JR, Gandhi S, Dick-Onuoha S, Lewis A, El-Serag HB. The association between Barrett's esophagus and helicobacter pylori infection: a meta-analysis. Helicobacter. 2012;17(3):163–75.

51. Abe Y, Koike T, Iijima K, Imatani A, Ishida K, Yuki T, et al. Esophageal adenocarcinoma developing after eradication of helicobacter pylori. Case Rep Gastroenterol. 2011;5(2):355–60.
52. Abe Y, Iijima K, Koike T, Asanuma K, Imatani A, Ohara S, et al. Barrett's esophagus is characterized by the absence of helicobacter pylori infection and high levels of serum pepsinogen I concentration in Japan. J Gastroenterol Hepatol. 2009;24(1):129–34.
53. Ho KY, Chan YH, Kang JY. Increasing trend of reflux esophagitis and decreasing trend of helicobacter pylori infection in patients from a multiethnic Asian country. Am J Gastroenterol. 2005;100:1923–8.
54. Rajendra S, Ackroyd R, Robertson IK, Ho JJ, Karim N, Kutty KM. Helicobacter pylori, ethnicity, and the gastroesophageal reflux disease spectrum: a study from the East. Helicobacter. 2007;12:177–83.
55. Fernandes ML, Seow A, Chan YH, Ho KY. Opposing trends in incidence of esophageal squamous cell carcinoma and adenocarcinoma in a multi-ethnic Asian country. Am J Gastroenterol. 2006;101(7):1430–6.
56. Yee YK, Cheung TK, Chan AO, Yuen MF, Wong BC. Decreasing trend of esophageal adenocarcinoma in Hong Kong. Cancer Epidemiol Biomark Prev. 2007;16(12):2637–40.
57. Chung JW, Lee GH, Choi KS, Kim DH, Jung KW, Song HJ, et al. Unchanging trend of esophagogastric junction adenocarcinoma in Korea: experience at a single institution based on Siewert's classification. Dis Esophagus. 2009;22(8):676–81.
58. Lu CL, Lang HC, Luo JC, Liu CC, Lin HC, Chang FY, et al. Increasing trend of the incidence of esophageal squamous cell carcinoma, but not adenocarcinoma, in Taiwan. Cancer Causes Control. 2010;21(2):269–74.
59. Hvid-Jensen F, Pedersen L, Drewes AM, Sørensen HT, Funch-Jensen P. Incidence of adenocarcinoma among patients with Barrett's esophagus. N Engl J Med. 2011;365(15):1375–83.
60. Lee SY, Yasuda K, Yasuda I, Ho LKY, Ahn SY, Lee TY, et al. Different managements for esophageal epithelial neoplasms between the Japanese, Singaporean, and Korean endoscopists. Korean J Helicobacter Upper Gastrointest Res. 2011;11(1):59–64.

Extra-esophageal GERD: Myth or Reality?

11

Somchai Leelakusolvong, Ratha-korn Vilaichone, and Varocha Mahachai

Abstract

Extra-esophageal manifestations of gastroesophageal reflux (GERD) consist of many syndromes such as laryngitis, laryngopharyngeal reflux, asthma, chronic cough, chest pain, and dental erosion. Due to the lack of disease definition, the prevalence of these extra-esophageal syndromes is not precisely known. They may or may not be associated with typical symptoms of GERD. Since there is no gold standard for the diagnosis of extra-esophageal GERD, its diagnosis and management is challenging. The management of extra-esophageal GERD is often empiric and targeted at specific symptoms. The initial approach is to use empirical therapy with high-dose proton pump inhibitors (PPIs), and further investigations are required in unresponsive cases. The continuation of PPI therapy is not recommended in patients who do not respond to empiric therapy with PPI.

Keywords

Extra-esophageal • GERD • pH monitoring • Asthma • Esophagitis • Laryngitis

S. Leelakusolvong
Gastrointestinal Division, Department of Medicine, Siriraj Hospital,
Prannok Road, Bangkok, Thailand

R.-k. Vilaichone
Gastrointestinal Unit, Department of Medicine, Thammasat University Hospital,
Pathumthani, Thailand

V. Mahachai (✉)
Department of Gastroenterology, Chulalongkorn University,
Ramma 4 Road, Bangkok, Thailand
e-mail: vmahachai@btinternet.com

© Springer India 2018
P. Sharma et al. (eds.), *The Rise of Acid Reflux in Asia*,
DOI 10.1007/978-81-322-0846-4_11

139

Epidemiology

The prevalence of extra-esophageal GERD is not precisely known due to the lack of clarity in disease definition. Extra-esophageal symptoms of GERD can occur in patients with or without typical GERD symptoms. A study from the United States [1–3] demonstrated that pneumonia and noncardiac chest pain (NCCP) (23.6 and 23.1 %, respectively) had the highest prevalence, followed by hoarseness (14.8 %), bronchitis (14.0 %), dysphagia (13.5 %), dyspepsia (10.6 %), asthma (9.3 %), and globus sensation (7.0 %). Nearly half the patients with NCCP had symptoms for more than 5 years [3].

Another large population-based study found that patients with reflux esophagitis were more commonly associated with pharyngeal, laryngeal, chest, and sinus problems than other hospitalized controls [4]. Interestingly, erosive esophagitis was found to be an independent risk factor for sinusitis, pharyngitis, hoarseness, laryngeal diseases, chronic bronchitis, and pulmonary diseases [4]. In this study, nearly one-fifth of patients with GERD had extra-esophageal manifestations, and patients with erosive esophagitis were at greater risk of having extra-esophageal symptoms than those without erosive esophagitis [4]. When ambulatory 24-h esophageal pH monitoring, barium esophagram, and upper endoscopy were done to evaluate the GERD patients with and without extra-esophageal symptoms, GERD was detected in nearly 3/4 of patients with chronic hoarseness, most patients with laryngeal stenosis [5] and asthma [6], and in some patients with chronic cough [7]. Upper GI endoscopy demonstrated esophagitis in 30–40 % of patients with asthma and 20 % of patients with laryngitis [8, 9].

Pathophysiology

The pathophysiology of extra-esophageal symptoms is not precisely known. GERD contributes to extra-esophageal symptoms by two possible mechanisms, including aspiration of gastric contents into extra-esophageal organs during reflux episodes and vagal-mediated mechanisms [10–14]. These mechanisms are key factors in the link between typical GERD and the atypical manifestations of extra-esophageal symptoms. GERD can be viewed as a cofactor in a multifactorial disease process rather than the sole etiologic agent. Reflux of gastroduodenal contents into the esophagus and pharynx could induce cough by direct pharyngeal and laryngeal irritation, and aspiration causes tracheobronchial cough. Chronic cough can also be triggered by a vagal-mediated tracheal and bronchial reflex [15, 16]. Previous studies have demonstrated that the esophagus and bronchus share a vagus nerve innervation. Pressure differences between the abdominal and thorax at the time of coughing may cause repeated reflux and cough [16, 17].

Both aspiration of gastric contents into extra-esophageal organs and vagal-mediated mechanisms have been suggested for their roles in extra-esophageal symptoms of GERD by demonstrating the effects of esophageal acid on extra-esophageal organs. Dual-probe esophageal pH monitoring supports the role of reflux, and ambulatory pH studies have shown that acid reflux started from the proximal esophagus [18]. Physiologic protection prevents the entry of esophageal refluxate into the pharynx and larynx. Disturbance of these protective mechanisms may be responsible for the extra-esophageal GERD manifestations. Acid reflux into the esophagus may irritate the receptors in the distal esophagus, causing noncardiac chest discomfort [19].

Reflex actions of the trachea protect the airway during burping and regurgitation. In addition, esophago-glottal reflux provides protection to the pharynx and respiratory tract from refluxate by closure of the vocal cords and forward movement of the glottis [18]. Swallowing mechanism plays an important role in preventing reflux through the upper esophageal sphincter [19]. Stimulation of the pharynx by fluids and a clean pharyngeal area induces closure of the glottis. The pharyngeal and laryngeal reflex mechanisms serve as important mechanisms in reducing aspiration and enhancing pharyngeal clearance by inducing cough reflex and mucociliary action of the bronchus and trachea [18].

Clinical Manifestations of Extra-esophageal GERD

The Montreal definition of GERD includes a wide spectrum of esophageal and extra-esophageal symptoms. Extra-esophageal symptoms that have established association with GERD include chronic cough, noncardiac chest pain, bronchial asthma, laryngopharyngeal symptoms, dental erosions, hoarseness, globus sensation, sore throat, vocal cord inflammation, aspiration, pulmonary fibrosis, pneumonia, and sleep disturbances, as shown in Table 11.1 [20]. Other conditions that are possibly related to GERD are sinusitis, otitis media, and laryngeal nodules. Reflux-related cough, asthma, and laryngitis are the most frequently encountered extra-esophageal syndromes. The common extra-esophageal GERD manifestations are discussed in detail below.

Table 11.1 Extra-esophageal manifestations of GERD

Pulmonary	Pharyngo-laryngeal
Asthma	Pharyngitis
Aspiration pneumonia	Vocal cord granulomas
Chronic bronchitis	Subglottic stenosis
Bronchiectasis	Laryngitis
Interstitial pulmonary fibrosis	Stridor
Oral	Hoarseness
Halitosis	Globus
Dental caries	Laryngeal cancer
Poor oral hygiene	Chronic cough

Chronic Cough

GERD is one of the important causes of chronic cough. Chronic cough could be defined as cough longer than 8 weeks [21, 22]. A few common causes of chronic cough include postnasal drip syndrome (PNDS), asthma, and the use of ACE inhibitors. Gastric refluxate can trigger chronic cough by irritation of the upper airway, by aspiration, and by stimulating esophagobronchial reflex, thereby stimulating sensory nerve receptors [17]. An increase in intra-abdominal pressure during cough induces the passage of refluxate through the lower esophageal sphincter [23, 24]. Reflux-associated cough correlates better with distal than proximal esophageal acid exposure, and esophagobronchial reflex is activated by a smaller amount of acid reflux. Recent studies have shown a relationship between reflux events and episodes of coughing. One study has demonstrated that even most of cough symptoms did not suddenly follow reflux events, where one-third of patients cough within 2 min of a reflux [27]. Chronic cough may be caused by micro-aspiration, resulting in stimulation of laryngeal and tracheobronchial cough receptors, although the evidence to support this is limited. Some patients with chronic cough from GERD may not have typical GERD symptoms. A study has shown that only a minority of patients with cough secondary to GERD had evidence of esophagitis on endoscopy [25]. Another study [26] found that only a small number of cough symptoms were related to hypopharyngeal reflux.

Noncardiac Chest Pain (NCCP)

NCCP often presents as angina-like chest pain in patients without organic heart disease [28, 29]. GERD is a well-known cause of noncardiac chest pain [28]. Heartburn can be documented in 10–70% of the patients [20]. Cardiac chest pain and chest pain from GERD likely share the same presentations. In a study by Locke et al., noncardiac chest pain was reported in 37% of patients with frequent heartburn symptoms, compared to 7.9% of patients reporting no GERD symptoms [29], but cardiac and esophageal motility disorders have to be excluded. The response mechanism likely can be explained by refluxate of gastroduodenal content, e.g., gastric acid and pepsin into esophageal mucosa, which stimulate the vagus nerve and finally cause the symptoms [30, 31]. The Neuro-Enteric Clinical Research Group from the United States demonstrated that only a small number of patients with NCCP had evidence of mucosal erosions on upper GI endoscopy [32]. Diagnostic testing for esophageal motility, ambulatory pH, and impedance monitoring is usually preserved for patients who do not respond to an empiric trial of PPI therapy [33].

Bronchial Asthma

Bronchial asthma has a strong association with GERD based on both epidemiologic studies and physiologic testing with ambulatory 24-h pH monitoring [34, 35]. Studies have also demonstrated high prevalence of GERD in asthmatic patients [36] and it is estimated to be between 34 and 89% [37]. GERD could induce bronchial asthma by the vagal-mediated and aspiration mechanisms.

GERD is highly prevalent in asthmatic patients who may or may not have reflux symptoms. Esophageal acid perfusion can induce airway reactivity, and micro-aspiration can cause airway constriction or can increase airway reactivity as a result of chronic inflammation. Bronchoconstriction in asthma can increase TLESR, causing reflux. Asthma and reflux have bidirectional interaction that potentially leads to a self-perpetuating vicious cycle. Heartburn and regurgitation before an asthma attack, or asthma symptoms occurring after meals, should be highly suspicious of being a result of GERD.

A high prevalence of esophageal motility diseases has been documented in patients with asthma. Pulmonary symptoms and pulmonary function in patients who have received acid-suppressive treatment have better outcomes [38]. Meier et al. evaluated pulmonary function of asthma patients treated with 20 mg of omeprazole twice a day for 6 weeks and demonstrated that 27% of patients with GERD had increase in FEV1 after treatment [39]. Sontag et al. [38] have evaluated the effect of H2-blockers and fundoplication in patients with both GERD and asthma. Surgical patients had a significant improvement in nighttime attacks compared to those who received H2-blockers or controls after a 2-year follow-up. Furthermore, they also had significant improvement in mean asthma symptom scores compared to those who received medical treatment or controls. Similarly, in a randomized controlled trial by the American Lung Association Asthma Clinical Research Center, it was found that among 412 patients with poor asthma control to either esomeprazole 40 mg twice daily or placebo control, there was higher benefit of PPI therapy in asthmatic patients than in the control group [40]. However, a Cochrane review of GERD treatment in asthma demonstrated only minimal improvement of asthma symptoms with anti-reflux treatment [41].

Laryngopharyngeal Symptoms

GERD is one of the important causes of laryngeal inflammation [42]. Common symptoms well known as laryngopharyngeal reflux (LPR) include globus, hoarseness, sore throat, cough, frequent throat clearance, dysphagia, and odynophagia. These symptoms are not specific and could be seen in patients with allergies to pollen, cigarette smoke, etc. [43]. However, GERD should be suspected in patients who have a long duration of symptoms and a history of laryngeal inflammation, as half of the patients with otolaryngologic manifestations [5] have classic reflux symptoms. The most common laryngeal findings noted with GERD are erythema and edema of the cricoarytenoid folds and the posterior aspects of vocal cords, which are the hypopharyngeal regions closest to the proximal esophagus [44]. Laryngoscopic findings of LPR are, however, nonspecific and can be found in healthy volunteers and may also be associated with smoking, alcohol, postnatal drip, and certain medications. More than 50% of patients with throat symptoms due to acid reflux have normal laryngoscopic findings. It is difficult to perform proximal pH monitoring because of its poor reproducibility. Combined pH impedance monitoring suggests that a majority of pharyngeal reflux for classic reflux symptoms in patients with otolaryngologic manifestations [5] are gaseous in nature.

Hoarseness caused by GERD occurs in approximately 10% of all cases. Globus sensation may be associated with GERD in up to half of cases [44]. Globus is defined as perception of a lump in the throat, regardless of swallowing, and frequently happens between meals and generally disappears at night or while eating. The etiology is still uncertain. More than half of patients with chronic laryngitis and sore throat have been diagnosed with acid reflux, which causes symptoms as well as erythema of the posterior vocal cords, contact ulceration, vocal cord polyps, granuloma formation, and subglottic stenosis among patients who have had prior endotracheal intubation [44].

Oral Manifestations

Oral manifestations of extra-esophageal GERD are prevalent in 5–97.5% of patients with GERD and include dental erosions, halitosis, water brash, mouth ulceration, taste disturbance, and glossodynia. Dental erosions occur due to intrinsic and extrinsic acid that exceed the buffering capacity of saliva, leading to clinical dissolution of enamel. GERD is observed in 21–83% of patients with dental erosions [45]. Early recognition of the role of GERD is key for prevention or treatment of dental erosions and other oral manifestations of extra-esophageal GERD.

Sleep Disturbances and GERD

Nocturnal reflux is associated with esophageal injury as well as a higher prevalence of laryngeal and pulmonary manifestations. GERD can affect the quality of sleep by awakening patients from sleep due to nocturnal heartburn, and reflux may result in amnestic arousals. Abnormal esophageal acid exposure is highly associated with obstructive sleep apnea [80%]. Studies have shown frequency of GERD attacks in patients with obstructive sleep apnea.

Other ENT Manifestations of GERD

Other ENT manifestations of extra-esophageal GERD include chronic rhinosinusitis, otitis media, subglottic stenosis, and laryngeal cancer. Nasopharyngeal exposure to reflux has been found in patients with rhinosinusitis. GERD treatment with PPI may improve the symptoms of sinusitis [46]. Extra-esophageal GERD may also be associated with otitis media, especially in infants. Subglottic stenosis secondary to reflux can occur in infants and adults. There is a strong association of positive pH studies showing acid reflux in these patients. GERD has been implicated as increasing the risk of laryngeal cancer, although the evidence to support their association is not definite [47].

Diagnosis and Treatment of Extra-esophageal GERD

There is significant controversy over how to diagnose extra-esophageal reflux syndromes such as reflux laryngitis or LPR, chronic cough, and asthma (Table 11.2), as there are no ideal and reliable tests. Other common non-GERD causes, such as suspected reflux laryngitis, should be excluded, and the patient should be evaluated by an ear, nose, and throat (ENT) physician. Those presenting with chronic cough should be evaluated by a pulmonologist [47].

Neither endoscopy nor pH is a gold standard in establishing an association between patients' symptoms from extra-esophageal syndromes and GERD. Appropriate diagnostic tools for each manifestation of extra-esophageal GERD are available, as shown in Table 11.2, but may not be cost-effective. The diagnosis and treatment of LPR, chronic cough, and asthma are discussed here.

Laryngopharyngeal Reflux (LPR)

The diagnosis and treatment of LPR remain controversial because of the lack of definite diagnostic criteria and treatment goals. Similar to the initial management of esophageal GERD, lifestyle modification (LSM) should be recommended to any extra-esophageal GERD patient, even though limited data are available to support the benefit of LSM in extra-esophageal GERD. The initial approach is empiric PPI treatment, even in the absence of typical GERD symptom or confirmation of GERD. However, studies have failed to show the benefit of PPIs over placebo in symptom improvement in suspected GERD-related chronic laryngitis. In unresponsive cases, causes other than GERD need to be excluded.

Table 11.2 Diagnostic testing for a suspected extra-esophageal GERD patient

Testing	Recommended tests for LPR/ chronic cough/asthma
Otolaryngologic symptom and sign score (RSIs/RFSs)	LPR
Salivary pepsin assay (pepsin test)	LPR/chronic cough/asthma
Laryngoscopy	LPR
Endoscopy (conventional and magnifying endoscopy ± chromoendoscopy)	LPR/chronic cough/asthma
Ambulatory pH monitoring (catheter based or bravo capsule) with/without impedance	LPR/chronic cough/asthma
Pharyngeal pH	LPR/chronic cough/asthma
Esophageal manometry or high-resolution manometry	LPR/chronic cough/asthma
PPI (PPI test)	LPR/chronic cough/asthma
Histology	LPR/chronic cough/asthma

Reflux Symptom Index (RSI), Reflux Finding Score (RFS), and Laryngoscopy

The clinical diagnosis of LPR is somewhat elusive, as the symptoms and signs are nonspecific and do not always correlate with reflux. RSI and RFS are self-administered assessments to document physical findings and symptom severity of LPR, although they have poor sensitivity and specificity for diagnosing LPR [48–51]. Laryngoscopic findings are not specific for reflux laryngitis, as similar findings can be found in healthy individuals, and have poor interobserver reliabilities. The finding of laryngitis may also be found in other non-GERD causes, including allergy, smoking, and voice abuse. Therefore, LPR should not be diagnosed based on laryngoscopic finding alone [48–52].

Pepsin Test

The pepsin salivary test is a rapid noninvasive test to detect salivary pepsin, which is a marker for detecting GERD. Detection of pepsin in the laryngopharynx suggests refluxate from the stomach. The presence of pepsin can be tested by the anti-human pepsin antibodies. Pepsin was present in 96% of laryngeal biopsy specimens taken from 19 patients with suspected LPR, while pepsin was not detected in any control subjects [53]. Sensitivity and specificity of the pepsin test were found to be 87%, with a positive predictive value (PPV) of 81% and negative predictive value (NPV) of 78% by using a pepsin lateral flow device [54].

Another study has shown that the detection of pepsin in laryngeal mucosa by immunohistochemistry (IHC) to diagnose LPR has an 80% sensitivity and 85.7% specificity [55]. Another study using an enzymatic method to measure salivary/sputum pepsin in 16 GERD patients has shown the correlation between the mean proximal and distal esophageal pH values and salivary pepsin assay [56]. This pepsin test has sensitivity and specificity of 89% and 68%, respectively, based on the pH monitoring results [57].

In addition, the pepsin test can clearly document GERD and signs of LPR with good concordance between pepsin detection in biopsy and sputum specimens. Anti-reflux surgery is also successful in eradicating pepsin, and it seems to predict clinical improvement of LPR after surgery. The pepsin test is a fast and easy test for the detection of salivary pepsin, with acceptable sensitivity and specificity. Further studies are required to evaluate the usefulness of this test for diagnosing LPR [58].

Endoscopy

Esophagogastroduodenoscopy (EGD) is useful in visualizing the erosive esophagitis (EE) and Barrett's esophagus and for excluding the other esophageal mucosal disorders. The prevalence of EE in patients with suspected GERD-related ENT symptoms was shown to be between 10 and 63% [59]. Studies from Asian countries—Thailand, Turkey, and Malaysia—showed the prevalence of EE to be 9%, 11%, and 48%, respectively [60–62]. Interestingly, it was shown that using a magnifying narrow-band imaging (NBI) endoscope can increase the percentage of finding esophageal mucosal abnormality up to 62% with criteria of abnormal vascular pattern of esophageal mucosa, compared with 9% by conventional white light endoscope, suggesting that magnifying NBI endoscopy can be an important diagnostic tool in identifying esophageal mucosal abnormalities [60]. However, the correlation between these abnormal findings and clinical GERD-related LPR is not clear, and finding EE on endoscopy does not establish a diagnosis of GERD-related reflux laryngitis or other extra-esophageal GERD syndromes. The American College of Gastroenterology (ACG) guidelines do not recommend the upper endoscopy for establishing a diagnosis of extra-esophageal GERD syndromes [48].

Ambulatory pH Monitoring

Ambulatory pH monitoring is considered a useful test for the diagnosis of extra-esophageal GERD disorders, as it documents a pathological gastroesophageal reflux.

The total percentage of time the pH is <4 is recommended as a parameter to discriminate physiological from pathological reflux [63]. There is a great variability in the prevalence of abnormal pH monitoring in patients with laryngitis, [64] asthma [65], and chronic cough [66]. Prevalence of LPR with abnormal pH monitoring from 14 studies from Western and Asian countries ranges from 18% to 100%, with an average of 53% [67]. When 24-h pH study is done, it has a 69% reproducibility, suggesting that a 24-h testing period may be too short a sampling period to accurately estimate reflux events [68]. However, there is no pH predictor of treatment response in LPR, and the false negative rate is as high as 30%, which are the limitations of this test. Evidence of pathological reflux on ambulatory monitoring does not establish GERD as the cause of the extra-esophageal symptoms. Meanwhile, a negative pH monitoring test should suggest the non-GERD causes. Additional impedance system to conventional pH catheter has been shown to give more information in regard to nonacid, gas, and liquid reflux. Furthermore, two additional indices in the interpretation of ambulatory pH monitoring are symptom index (SI) and the symptom-associated probability (SAP), although these two symptom indices could not be relied upon for GERD association [69, 70]. The sensitivity and specificity of symptom association analysis are limited, and there are no outcome studies to support using these parameters to monitor the treatment response in extra-esophageal GERD.

The pH monitoring off PPI therapy provides the baseline for reflux information, especially in patients with a low pretest likelihood of GERD, while an impedance pH monitoring may be useful in patients who are on PPI therapy and continue to have symptoms, or for those who have a high pretest likelihood of GERD [64, 71]. In addition, the new device for detecting the pharyngeal pH (ResTech®) showed a significantly higher number of reflux events in LPR patients compared with GERD patients and healthy volunteers, suggesting this test might have a role for the evaluation of suspected LPR patients with a faster detection rate and faster time to equilibrium pH [72].

Drug Therapy

Treatment of extra-esophageal GERD is often empirical and targeted at specific symptoms. Drug therapy for reflux laryngitis includes antisecretory agents such as proton pump inhibitors (PPIs), H_2 receptor antagonists (H_2RAs), and antacid. Other medications such as mucosal protective agents and transient lower esophageal sphincter relaxation (TLESR) reducer can also provide additional benefits. Evidence for the effectiveness of drug therapy is relatively weak. Guidelines of the American Gastroenterological Association and American College of Gastroenterology recommend PPI in patients with extra-esophageal GERD who also have typical symptoms of GERD or objective evidence of GERD by endoscopy or pH monitoring [48, 73].

Proton Pump Inhibitors (PPIs)

PPIs are the mainstay in the treatment of suspected LPR patients and can be given empirically. Response rate of PPI treatment ranges from 47 to 90% from the two open-labeled studies [74, 75]. A multicenter trial failed to show significant difference in the resolution of symptoms or laryngeal signs of LPR between patients treated with high-dose esomeprazole and placebo for 16 weeks [76]. Interestingly, a meta-analysis from eight randomized placebo-controlled trials in LPR has demonstrated an absolute rate of PPI response of 50%, while the placebo response was 41%. This study suggested that PPI treatment in suspected GERD-related LPR was not significantly better than placebo treatment [77]. No significant difference in symptom resolution between PPI for 2–4 months and placebo was demonstrated in other randomized controlled trials [72, 76, 78]. The subgroups of patients responded to PPI treatment included patients with moderate to severe reflux parameters at baseline, moderate-sized (larger than 4 cm) hiatal hernia, and concomitant heartburn and/or regurgitation in addition to their LPR symptoms [71].

A suspected LPR patient should initially be treated with empirical PPI therapy for the duration of 1–2 months (Fig. 11.1). If symptoms improve, PPI should be continued up to 6 months to allow healing of the laryngeal tissue [79], after which the dose should be tapered to minimal acid suppression. However, there are limited data from Asian and Western clinical trials to guide the duration of treatment.

H2 Receptor Antagonists (H₂RAs)

H_2RAs in LPR may play a role in controlling nocturnal acid breakthrough (NAB). A meta-analysis from eight small randomized controlled trials (n = 58 in H_2RA group and n = 58 in control group) has shown that additional bedtime H_2RA can decrease the prevalence rate of NAB and decrease the percentage of time during which intragastric pH is less than 4. However, the use of nighttime H2 RAs in LPR has not proven to be beneficial [80, 81]. However, another open-labeled prospective cohort study in 30 patients receiving additional ranitidine 300 mg, with omeprazole 20 mg twice daily, compared with other PPI twice a day, did not show any difference in the treatment response, suggesting that adding H_2RAs in NAB does not improve the symptom response in LPR patients [80].

Surgical Fundoplication

Laparoscopic fundoplication failed to improve laryngeal symptoms at 1-year post-surgery in 25 suspected LPR patients unresponsive to initial PPI therapy, despite physiologic control of all reflux events [82]. A retrospective cohort study in 237

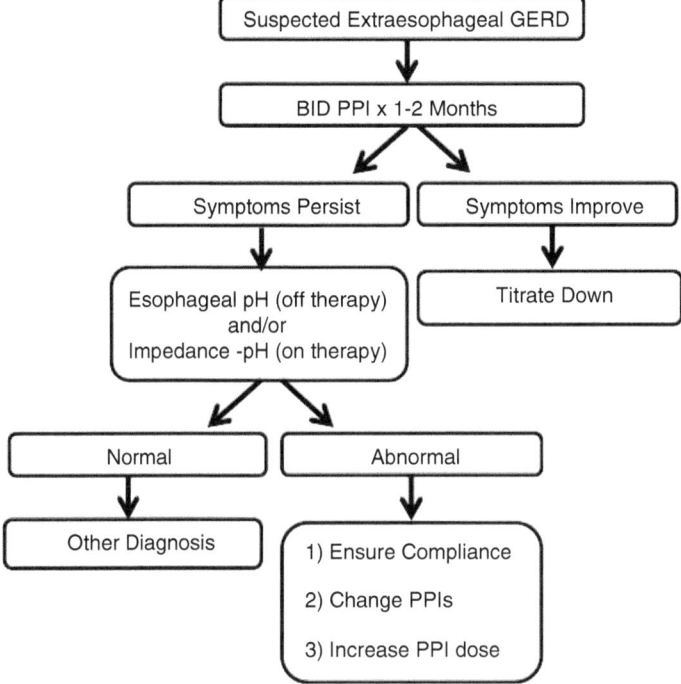

Fig. 11.1 Diagnosis and treatment algorithm for extra-esophageal reflux

patients showed that both heartburn with or without regurgitation and esophageal pH < 4 more than 12% of a 24-h period predicted post-fundoplication resolution of the presenting extra-esophageal reflux symptom [83]. The ACG guidelines do not recommend fundoplication for patients who are unresponsive to aggressive medical anti-reflux therapy [48].

Chronic Cough

It is estimated that up to 75% of patients with GERD-related cough do not have classical GERD symptoms, which makes this diagnosis challenging. Besides, GERD can coexist in patients with cough due to other conditions. The common non-GERD causes for chronic cough must be excluded before establishing the diagnosis of GERD-related chronic cough, such as history of taking angiotensin-converting enzyme inhibitor (ACEI), postnasal drip syndrome (PNDS), asthma, and chronic bronchitis. The investigations for GERD-related chronic cough are similar to those in reflux laryngitis (Table 11.2).

Diagnostic Tests

Tests for diagnosing GERD-related cough include EGD, ambulatory pH monitoring, and PPI test. There is poor correlation between endoscopic finding, symptoms, and results of pH study. Previous study has shown that out of 45 patients with chronic cough, 55% reported classical reflux symptoms, but only 15.5% had endoscopy-proven esophagitis [25]. Similar to LPR, most patients with GERD-related cough will have normal endoscopic findings. Ambulatory pH monitoring has a sensitivity, at best, of 90% and specificity as low as 66% [84]. A 24-h pH study with cough correlation may be useful to diagnose GERD-related cough, but it has low positive predictive value and can be misleading. A previous study showed that pH monitoring is not a reliable predictor of acid reflux-induced chronic cough because only 35% of patients with abnormal pH meter responded to high-dose omeprazole [21].

Management

The strategy in the management of GERD-related chronic cough is similar to that of reflux laryngitis. Lifestyle modification should be an initial approach. A study on empirical PPI therapy in 214 patients with chronic cough over a 3.5-year period showed that 79% of patients experienced symptom improvement after empirical of PPI treatment [85]. It is therefore recommended to give an empirical trial with PPIs for 1–3 months in patients with GERD symptoms or those likely to have silent GERD. Fundoplication may be recommended for those patients who have GERD-related cough that previously responded to PPI therapy. PPI twice daily is a drug of choice. Nevertheless, recent meta-analysis of nine placebo-controlled studies has shown insufficient evidence in favor of PPI therapy (OR 0.46; 95% CI, 0.19–1.15). Two studies showed improvement in cough after 5 days to 2 weeks of treatment [86]. A short course of PPI therapy may be a reasonable initial approach for GERD-related cough. The non-PPI therapy for GERD-associated cough with H_2Ras and prokinetic agents was not found to be useful, and there has not been evidence to support the benefit of fundoplication. Patients who responded to surgical intervention may be those who responded to medical therapy for typical symptoms of GERD [42].

In summary, the treatment of GERD-associated cough should begin with a short course of empirical PPI therapy after excluding the other common non-GERD causes (Fig. 11.1). The investigations should be considered in those who remain symptomatic to exclude the non-GERD causes or the reflux-causing chronic cough from the residual acid or nonacid reflux. Other medications and fundoplication should be reserved for those who partially responded to the PPI treatment with evidence of acid reflux after 24-h pH monitoring with typical reflux symptoms.

Reflux Asthma

GERD-related asthma should be suspected in any patient who presents with adult-onset asthma, poor control of asthma, worsening asthma symptoms related to large meals, and onset of heartburn or regurgitation before asthma attacks [87].

Diagnostic Tests

The prevalence of asthma in individuals with GERD was 4.6%, whereas in controls was 3.9% [19]. Studies from Asian countries have shown that the prevalence of reflux esophagitis was between 27.8 and 39.3%. In addition, the prevalence of GERD in asthmatic Asian patients was 6.5–44% compared to 0.6–19.4% in the control group [88]. The prevalence of GERD is high in the asthmatic patients, with low prevalence of typical reflux symptoms [34].

There is no diagnostic test that can identify anti-reflux-responsive asthma. An empirical trial of twice-daily PPIs for 3 months is recommended in asthma patients with GERD symptoms. Esophageal pH study may be useful to correlate asthma symptoms with GERD, to diagnose silent GERD, and to assess the adequacy of acid suppression.

Management

The benefit of PPI for GERD-associated asthma is still conflicting. Previous systematic reviews on anti-reflux treatment including PPI, H_2RA, and surgery in GERD-related asthma have shown that anti-reflux treatment did not consistently improve lung function, asthma symptoms, nocturnal asthma, or the use of asthma medications [89]. High-dose esomeprazole given to asthma patients for 4 months has been shown to improve peak expiratory flow (PEF) [90]. The improvements of pulmonary functions are, however, inconsistent after a high dose of PPI [91, 92]. Another study failed to show the benefit of high-dose lansoprazole given for 24 weeks in reducing daily asthma symptoms and improving pulmonary function [92].

In summary, the benefit of anti-reflux therapy in GERD-associated asthma is inconsistent. Behavioral and lifestyle modification should be implemented in asthma patients with GERD symptoms. Fundoplication should be reserved for those patients who have asthma improvement with GERD therapy.

Summary

Extra-esophageal GERD syndromes include reflux laryngitis, chronic cough, asthma, and dental erosions, whereas reflux chest pain and typical reflux syndrome have been classified as symptomatic syndrome of GERD [10]. Due to limited data from Asian countries, the prevalence of extra-esophageal GERD in Asia is not exactly known, although the overall GERD prevalence is much lower than that in the Western countries. Pathogenesis of these syndromes is still not clearly understood, and it is proposed to be a multifactorial process.

Nonetheless, a majority of the extra-esophageal GERD patients do not present with the typical GERD symptoms. Investigations such as upper endoscopy and ambulatory pH monitoring have low sensitivity and specificity and are considered not cost-effective. The empirical PPI therapy is the most cost-effective approach and is considered to be a first-line therapy in the management of extra-esophageal GERD. Additional therapy beyond PPI requires further confirmation of its benefit before it can be recommended in the management of extra-esophageal GERD.

In those patients who fail to respond or partially respond to PPI, ambulatory pH monitoring and/or impedance pH monitoring can be considered to document if the pathological reflux causes the extra-esophageal symptoms. Other non-GERD causes should be evaluated according to the specific syndromes. Surgical fundoplication should not be considered in patients who are unresponsive to aggressive PPI therapy. Fundoplication may be beneficial in patients who respond to antisecretory agents, who present with typical GERD symptoms, and those with large hiatal hernia.

References

1. Dent J, El-Serag HB, Wallander MA, Johansson S. Epidemiology of gastro-oesophageal reflux disease: a systematic review. Gut. 2005;54:710–7. doi:10.1136/gut.2004.051821. PMID: 15831922
2. Mahachai V, Vilaichone RK. Current status of helicobacter pylori infection in Thailand. Helicobacter Res. 2011;5(3):38–44.
3. Locke GR III, Talley NJ, Fett SL, Zinsmeister AR, Melton LJ III. Prevalence and clinical spectrum of gastro-esophageal reflux: a population-based study in Olmsted County. Minnesota Gastroenterology. 1997;112:1448–56.
4. El-Serag HB, Sonnenberg A. Comorbid occurrence of laryngeal or pulmonary disease with esophagitis in United States military veterans. Gastroenterology. 1997;113:755–60.
5. Koufman JA. The otolaryngologic manifestations of gastroesophageal reflux disease (GERD). A clinical investigation of 225 patients using ambulatory 24-hour monitoring and an experimental investigation of the role of acid and pepsin in the development of laryngeal injury. Laryngoscope. 1991;101:1–78.
6. Sontag SJ, O'Connell S, Khandelwal S, Miller T, Nemchausky B, Schnell TG, et al. Most asthmatics have gastroesophageal reflux with or without bronchodilator therapy. Gastroenterology. 1990;99(3):613–20.
7. Irwin RS, Curley FJ, French CL. Difficult to control asthma. Contributing factors and outcome of a systematic management protocol. Chest. 1993;103:1662–9.
8. Larrain A, Carrasco E, Galleguillos F, Sepulveda R, Pope CE 2nd. Medical and surgical treatment of nonallergic asthma associated with gastroesophageal reflux. Chest. 1991;99(6):1330–5.
9. Sontag SJ, Schnell TG, Miller TQ, Khandelwal S, O'Connell S, Chejfec G, et al. Prevalence of oesophagitis in asthmatics. Gut. 1992;33(7):872–6.
10. Vakil N, van Zanten SV, Kahrilas P, Dent J, Jones R. The Montreal definition and classification of gastroesophageal reflux disease: a global evidence-based consensus. Am J Gastroenterol. 2006;101(8):1900–20. quiz 43
11. Field SK, Evans JA, Price LM. The effects of acid perfusion of the esophagus on ventilation and respiratory sensation. Am J Respir Crit Care Med. 1998;157(4 Pt 1):1058–62.
12. Ing AJ, Ngu MC, Breslin AB. Pathogenesis of chronic persistent cough associated with gastroesophageal reflux. Am J Respir Crit Care Med. 1994;149(1):160–7.
13. Adhami T, Goldblum JR, Richter JE, Vaezi MF. The role of gastric and duodenal agents in laryngeal injury: an experimental canine model. Am J Gastroenterol. 2004;99(11):2098–106.
14. Tuchman DN, Boyle JT, Pack AI, Scwartz J, Kokonos M, Spitzer AR, et al. Comparison of airway responses following tracheal or esophageal acidification in the cat. Gastroenterology. 1984;87(4):872–81.
15. Stanghellini V. Relationship between upper gastrointestinal symptoms and lifestyle, psychosocial factors and comorbidity in the general population: results from the domestic/international gastroenterology surveillance study (DIGEST). Scand J Gastroenterol Suppl. 1999;231:29–37.

16. Poe RH, Kallay MC. Chronic cough and gastroesophageal reflux disease:experience with specific therapy for diagnosis and treatment. Chest. 2003;123(3):679–84.
17. Irwin RS. Chronic cough due to gastroesophageal reflux disease: ACCP evidence-based clinical practice guidelines. Chest. 2006;129(1 Suppl):80S–94S.
18. Hogan WJ, Shaker R. Supraesophageal complications of gastroesophageal reflux. Dis Mon. 2000;46(3):195–232.
19. Fennerty MB. Extraesophageal gastroesophageal reflux disease: presentations and approach to treatment. Gastroenterol Clin. 1999;28:861–73.
20. Fass R. Extraesophageal manifestation of GERD. AGA Postgraduate Course AGA. 2007:23–9.
21. Ours TM, Kavuru MS, Schilz RJ, Richter JE. A prospective evaluation of esophageal testing and a double-blind, randomized study of omeprazole in a diagnostic and therapeutic algorithm for chronic cough. Am J Gastroenterol. 1999;94(11):3131–8. Epub 1999 Nov 24
22. Schappert SM. National ambulatory medical care survey, 1991: summary. In: Vitals and Health Statistics No 230. Washington, DC: US Dept of Health and Human Services; 1993. p. 1–20.
23. Ing AJ, Ngu MC, Breslin AB. Pathogenesis of chronic persistent cough associated with gastroesophageal reflux. Am J Respir Crit Care. 1994;149:160–7.
24. Smith J, Woodcock A. New developments in the objective assessment of cough. Lung. 2008;186(Suppl 1):S48–54.
25. Baldi F, Cappiello R, Cavoli C, Ghersi S, Torresan F, Roda E. Proton pump inhibitor treatment of patients with gastroesophageal reflux-related chronic cough: a comparison between two different daily doses of lansoprazole. World J Gastroenterol. 2006;12(1):82–8. Epub 2006 Jan 28
26. Patterson WG, Murat BW. Combined ambulatory esophageal manometry and dual-probe pH-metry in evaluation of patients with chronic unexplained cough. Dig Dis Sci. 1994;39:1117–25.
27. Sifrim D, Dupont L, Blondeau K, Zhang X, Tack J, Janssens J. Weakly acidic reflux in patients with chronic unexplained cough during 24 hour pressure, pH, and impedance monitoring. Gut. 2005;54(4):449–54.
28. Fass R, Navarro-Rodriguez T. Noncardiac chest pain. J Clin Gastroenterol. 2008;42(5):636–46.
29. Fang J, Bjorkman D. A critical approach to noncardiac chest pain: pathophysiology, diagnosis, and treatment. Am J Gastroenterol. 2001;96(4):958–68.
30. Parsons JP, Mastronade JG. Gastroesophageal reflux disease and asthma. Curr Opin Pulm Med. 2010;16:60–3.
31. American Lung Association Asthma Clinical Research Centers, Mastronarde JG, Anthonisen NR, Castro M, Holbrook JT, Leone FT, et al. Efficacy of esomeprazole for treatment of poorly controlled asthma. N Engl J Med. 2009;360(15):1487–99.
32. Hicks DM, Ours TM, Alelson TI, Vaezi MF, Richter JE. The prevalence of hypopharynx findings associated with gastroesophageal reflux in normal volunteers. J Voice. 2002;16(4):564–79.
33. Moore JM, Vaezi MF. Extraesophageal manifestations of gastroesophageal reflux disease: real or imagined? Curr Opin Gastroenterol. 2010;26:389–94.
34. Kiljander TO, Salomaa ER, Hietanen EK, Terho EO. Gastroesophageal reflux in asthmatics: a double-blind, placebo-controlled crossover study with omeprazole. Chest. 1999;116(5):1257–64. Epub 1999 Nov 13
35. Ahmed T, Vaezi MF. The role of pH monitoring in extraesophageal gastroesophageal reflux disease. Gastrointest Endosc Clin N Am. 2005;15(2):319–31.
36. American Lung Association. Prevalence based on revised National Health Interview Survey. Available at: www.lungusa.org/data/data_102000.html. Accessed 16 Jan 2003.
37. Harding SM, Richter JE. The role of gastroesophageal reflux in chronic cough and asthma. Chest. 1997;111:1389–402.
38. Sontag SJ, O'Connell S, Khandelwal S, Greenlee H, Schnell T, Nemchausky B, et al. Asthmatics with gastroesophageal reflux: long term results of a randomized trial of medical and surgical antireflux therapies. Am J Gastroenterol. 2003;98(5):987–99.
39. Meier JH, McNally PR, Punja M, Freeman SR, Sudduth RH, Stocker N, et al. Does omeprazole (Prilosec) improve respiratory function in asthmatics with gastroesophageal reflux? A double-blind, placebo-con-trolled crossover study. Dig Dis Sci. 1994;39(10):2127–33.

40. Mastronarde JG, Anthonisen NR, Castro M, Holbrook JT, Leone FT, Teague WG, et al. Efficacy of esomeprazole for treatment of poorly controlled asthma. N Engl J Med. 2009;360(15):1487–99.
41. Gibson PG, Powell H, Coughlan J, Wilson AJ, Hensley MJ, Abramson M, et al. Limited (information only) patient education programs for adults with asthma. Cochrane Database Syst Rev. 2002;2:CD001005. Epub 2002 Jun 22
42. Vaezi MF. Laryngitis and gastroesophageal reflux disease: increasing prevalence or poor diagnostic tests? Am J Gastroenterol. 2004;99(5):786–8. Epub 2004 May 7
43. Diamond L. Laryngopharyngeal reflux – it's not GERD. JAAPA. 2005;18(8):50–3. Epub 2005 Aug 27
44. Ohman L, Olofsson J, Tibbling L, Ericsson G. Esophageal dysfunction in patients with contact ulcer of the larynx. Ann Otol Rhinol Laryngol. 1983;92(3 Pt 1):228–30.
45. Schroeder PL, Filler SJ, Ramirez B, Lazarchik DA, Vaezi MF, Richter JE. Dental erosion and acid reflux disease. Ann Intern Med. 1995;122(11):809–15.
46. Bothwell MR, Parsons DS, Talbot A, Barbero GJ, Wilder B. Outcome of reflux therapy on pediatric chronic sinusitis. Otolaryngol Head Neck Surg. 1999;121(3):255–62.
47. Wilson JA. What is the evidence that gastroesophageal reflux is involved in the etiology of laryngeal cancer? Curr Opin Qtolaryngol Head Neck Surg. 2005;13:97–100.
48. Katz PO, Gerson LB, Vela MF. Guidelines for the diagnosis and management of gastroesophageal reflux disease. Am J Gastroenterol. 2013;108(3):308–28. quiz 29. Epub 2013 Feb 20
49. Belafsky PC, Postma GN, Koufman JA. Validity and reliability of the reflux symptom index (RSI). J Voice. 2002;16(2):274–7. Epub 2002 Aug 2
50. Belafsky PC, Postma GN, Koufman JA. The validity and reliability of the reflux finding score (RFS). Laryngoscope. 2001;111(8):1313–7. Epub 2001 Sep 25
51. Park KH, Choi SM, Kwon SU, Yoon SW, Kim SU. Diagnosis of laryngopharyngeal reflux among globus patients. Otolaryngology. 2006;134(1):81–5. Epub 2006 Jan 10
52. Branski RC, Bhattacharyya N, Shapiro J. The reliability of the assessment of endoscopic laryngeal findings associated with laryngopharyngeal reflux disease. Laryngoscope. 2002;112(6):1019–24. Epub 2002 Aug 6
53. Johnston N, Knight J, Dettmar PW, Lively MO, Koufman J. Pepsin and carbonic anhydrase isoenzyme III as diagnostic markers for laryngopharyngeal reflux disease. Laryngoscope. 2004;114(12):2129–34. Epub 2004 Nov 27
54. Saritas Yuksel E, Hong SK, Strugala V, Slaughter JC, Goutte M, Garrett CG, et al. Rapid salivary pepsin test: blinded assessment of test performance in gastroesophageal reflux disease. Laryngoscope. 2012;122(6):1312–6. Epub 2012 Mar 27
55. Jiang A, Liang M, Su Z, Chai L, Lei W, Wang Z, et al. Immunohistochemical detection of pepsin in laryngeal mucosa for diagnosing laryngopharyngeal reflux. Laryngoscope. 2011;121(7):1426–30. Epub 2011 June 8
56. Potluri S, Friedenberg F, Parkman HP, Chang A, MacNeal R, Manus C, et al. Comparison of a salivary/sputum pepsin assay with 24-hour esophageal pH monitoring for detection of gastric reflux into the proximal esophagus, oropharynx, and lung. Dig Dis Sci. 2003;48(9):1813–7. Epub 2003 Oct 17
57. Kim TH, Lee KJ, Yeo M, Kim DK, Cho SW. Pepsin detection in the sputum/saliva for the diagnosis of gastroesophageal reflux disease in patients with clinically suspected atypical gastroesophageal reflux disease symptoms. Digestion. 2008;77(3–4):201–6. Epub 2008 Jul 12
58. Johnston N, Dettmar PW, Strugala V, Allen JE, Chan WW. Laryngopharyngeal reflux and GERD. Ann N Y Acad Sci. 2013;1300(1):71–9. Epub 2013/10/15
59. Poelmans J, Tack J. Extraoesophageal manifestations of gastro-oesophageal reflux. Gut. 2005;54(10):1492–9. Epub 2005 Sep 16
60. Sansak I, Leelakusolvong S, Prachayakul V, Pausawasdi N, Charatcharoenwitthaya P, Chainuvati S, et al. The usefulness of narrow band imaging system with magnifying endoscopy in evaluation of patients with laryngopharyngeal reflux disease. Gastroenterology. 2010;138(5):S1–S906.

61. Qua CS, Wong CH, Gopala K, Goh KL. Gastro-oesophageal reflux disease in chronic laryngitis: prevalence and response to acid-suppressive therapy. Aliment Pharmacol Ther. 2007;25(3):287–95. Epub 2007 Feb 3

62. Toros SZ, Toros AB, Yuksel OD, Ozel L, Akkaynak C, Naiboglu B. Association of laryngopharyngeal manifestations and gastroesophageal reflux. Eur Arch Otorhinolaryngol. 2009;266(3):403–9.

63. Pandolfino JE, Vela MF. Esophageal-reflux monitoring. Gastrointest Endosc. 2009;69(4):917–30.

64. Abou-Ismail A, Vaezi MF. Evaluation of patients with suspected laryngopharyngeal reflux: a practical approach. Curr Gastroenterol Rep. 2011;13(3):213–8. Epub 2011 March 02

65. Havemann BD, Henderson CA, El-Serag HB. The association between gastro-oesophageal reflux disease and asthma: a systematic review. Gut. 2007;56(12):1654–64. Epub 2007 Aug 08

66. Smith J, Woodcock A, Houghton L. New developments in reflux-associated cough. Lung. 2010;188(Suppl 1):S81–6. Epub 2009 Dec 22

67. Vaezi MF. Review article: the role of pH monitoring in extraoesophageal gastro-oesophageal reflux disease. Aliment Pharmacol Ther. 2006;23(Suppl 1):40–9. Epub 2006 Feb 18

68. Noordzij JP, Khidr A, Desper E, Meek RB, Reibel JF, Levine PA. Correlation of pH probe-measured laryngopharyngeal reflux with symptoms and signs of reflux laryngitis. Laryngoscope. 2002;112(12):2192–5. Epub 2002 Dec 04

69. Slaughter JC, Goutte M, Rymer JA, Oranu AC, Schneider JA, Garrett CG, et al. Caution about overinterpretation of symptom indexes in reflux monitoring for refractory gastroesophageal reflux disease. Clin Gastroenterol Hepatol. 2011;9(10):868–74. Epub 2011 July 26

70. Kavitt RT, Higginbotham T, Slaughter JC, Patel D, Yuksel ES, Lominadze Z, et al. Symptom reports are not reliable during ambulatory reflux monitoring. Am J Gastroenterol. 2012;107(12):1826–32. Epub 2012 Oct 24

71. Naik RD, Vaezi MF. Extra-esophageal manifestations of GERD: who responds to GERD therapy? Curr Gastroenterol Rep. 2013;15(4):318. Epub 2013 Feb 26

72. Steward DL, Wilson KM, Kelly DH, Patil MS, Schwartzbauer HR, Long JD, et al. Proton pump inhibitor therapy for chronic laryngo-pharyngitis: a randomized placebo-control trial. Otolaryngology. 2004;131(4):342–50. Epub 2004 Oct 07

73. Kahrilas PJ, Shaheen NJ, Vaezi MF. American Gastroenterological Association Institute technical review on the management of gastroesophageal reflux disease. Gastroenterology. 2008;135(4):1392–413, 413 e1–5. Epub 2008 Sep 20

74. Williams RB, Szczesniak MM, Maclean JC, Brake HM, Cole IE, Cook IJ. Predictors of outcome in an open label, therapeutic trial of high-dose omeprazole in laryngitis. Am J Gastroenterol. 2004;99(5):777–85. Epub 2004 May 07

75. Park W, Hicks DM, Khandwala F, Richter JE, Abelson TI, Milstein C, et al. Laryngopharyngeal reflux: prospective cohort study evaluating optimal dose of proton-pump inhibitor therapy and pretherapy predictors of response. Laryngoscope. 2005;115(7):1230–8. Epub 2005 Jul 5

76. Vaezi MF, Richter JE, Stasney CR, Spiegel JR, Iannuzzi RA, Crawley JA, et al. Treatment of chronic posterior laryngitis with esomeprazole. Laryngoscope. 2006;116(2):254–60. Epub 2006 Feb 10

77. Qadeer MA, Phillips CO, Lopez AR, Steward DL, Noordzij JP, Wo JM, et al. Proton pump inhibitor therapy for suspected GERD-related chronic laryngitis: a meta-analysis of randomized controlled trials. Am J Gastroenterol. 2006;101(11):2646–54. Epub 2006 Oct 14

78. Wo JM, Koopman J, Harrell SP, Parker K, Winstead W, Lentsch E. Double-blind, placebo-controlled trial with single-dose pantoprazole for laryngopharyngeal reflux. Am J Gastroenterol. 2006;101(9):1972–8. quiz 2169. Epub 2006 Sep 14

79. Koufman JA, Aviv JE, Casiano RR, Shaw GY. Laryngopharyngeal reflux: position statement of the committee on speech, voice, and swallowing disorders of the American Academy of Otolaryngology-Head and Neck Surgery. Otolaryngology. 2002;127(1):32–5. Epub 2002 Aug 6

80. Wang Y, Pan T, Wang Q, Guo Z. Additional bedtime H2-receptor antagonist for the control of nocturnal gastric acid breakthrough. Cochrane Database Syst Rev. 2009;4:CD004275. Epub 2009 Oct 13

81. McGlashan JA, Johnstone LM, Sykes J, Strugala V, Dettmar PW. The value of a liquid alginate suspension (Gaviscon Advance) in the management of laryngopharyngeal reflux. Eur Arch Otorhinolaryngol. 2009;266(2):243–51. Epub 2008/ May 29
82. Swoger J, Ponsky J, Hicks DM, Richter JE, Abelson TI, Milstein C, et al. Surgical fundoplication in laryngopharyngeal reflux unresponsive to aggressive acid suppression: a controlled study. Clin Gastroenterol Hepatol. 2006;4(4):433–41. Epub 2006 Apr 18
83. Francis DO, Goutte M, Slaughter JC, Garrett CG, Hagaman D, Holzman MD, et al. Traditional reflux parameters and not impedance monitoring predict outcome after fundoplication in extraesophageal reflux. Laryngoscope. 2011;121(9):1902–9. Epub 2011 Oct 26
84. Frye JW, Vaezi MF. Extraesophageal GERD. Gastroenterol Clin N Am. 2008;37(4):845–58, ix. Epub 2008 Nov 26
85. Poe RH, Kallay MC. Chronic cough and gastroesophageal reflux disease: experience with specific therapy for diagnosis and treatment. Chest. 2003;123(3):67984. Epub 2003 Mar 12
86. Chang AB, Lasserson TJ, Gaffney J, Connor FL, Garske LA. Gastro-oesophageal reflux treatment for prolonged non-specific cough in children and adults. Cochrane Database Syst Rev. 2011;1:CD004823. Epub 2011 Jan 21
87. Leggett JJ, Johnston BT, Mills M, Gamble J, Heaney LG. Prevalence of gastroesophageal reflux in difficult asthma: relationship to asthma outcome. Chest. 2005;127(4):1227–31. Epub 2005 Apr 12
88. Jung HK. Epidemiology of gastroesophageal reflux disease in Asia: a systematic review. Journal of neurogastroenterology and motility. 2011;17(1):14–27. Epub 2011 Mar 4
89. Gibson PG, Henry RL, Coughlan JL. Gastro-oesophageal reflux treatment for asthma in adults and children. Cochrane Database Syst Rev. 2003;2:CD001496. Epub 2003 Jun 14
90. Kiljander TO, Harding SM, Field SK, Stein MR, Nelson HS, Ekelund J, et al. Effects of esomeprazole 40 mg twice daily on asthma: a randomized placebo-controlled trial. Am J Resp Crit Care Med. 2006;173(10):1091–7. Epub 2005 Dec 17
91. Harding SM, Richter JE, Guzzo MR, Schan CA, Alexander RW, Bradley LA. Asthma and gastroesophageal reflux: acid suppressive therapy improves asthma outcome. Am J Med. 1996;100(4):395–405. Epub 1996 Apr 01
92. Littner MR, Leung FW, Ballard ED 2nd, Huang B, Samra NK. Effects of 24 weeks of lansoprazole therapy on asthma symptoms, exacerbations, quality of life, and pulmonary function in adult asthmatic patients with acid reflux symptoms. Chest. 2005;128(3):1128–35. Epub 2005 Sep 16

Hardik Parikh and Philip Abraham

Introduction

The Asian continent is the most diverse one with regard to ethnic groups, cultures, habits, and environment. Naturally, disease frequency and etiological factors will vary as widely. A condition such as gastroesophageal reflux disease (GERD) is dependent on diet and environment as much as on the individual and so is an archetypal case for study in such a situation.

GERD Prevalence in Asia

Population-based GERD prevalence data from the USA (28.8%) and Europe (23.7%) had showed significantly higher rates as compared to those in Asia [1]. Approximately 2.5–5% of Asians experience weekly heartburn and/or acid regurgitation [2]. There are substantial differences in GERD prevalence among Asian regions, but only East Asia shows rates consistently lower than 10% [3]. The prevalence is highest in West Asia (12.5–27.6%), less so in Central Asia (7.6–19.4%), and lowest in East Asia (2.5–9.4%) [3]. Rates ranging from 12.4% (Taiwan), 17% (Mainland China), to 29.8% (Hong Kong) have also been reported, though [4–9]. Rates reported from the Indian subcontinent (India, Bangladesh, and Pakistan) range from 7.6 to 24% [5, 6, 10]. The Asian Indian race (South Asia) seems to be at higher risk as compared to white Caucasians for developing GERD [11].

H. Parikh
Department of Gastroenterology, KEM Hospital and Seth GS Medical College,
Mumbai 400012, India

P. Abraham (✉)
Division of Gastroenterology, P.D. Hinduja Hospital,
VS Marg, Mahim, Mumbai 400016, India
e-mail: dr_pabraham@hindujahospital.com

© Springer India 2018
P. Sharma et al. (eds.), *The Rise of Acid Reflux in Asia*,
DOI 10.1007/978-81-322-0846-4_12

Ethnic differences in the prevalence of GERD within a region were studied in Singapore; a higher incidence was noted in Indians in Singapore (7.5%) as compared to Malays (3%) and Chinese (0.8%) [12]. Racial differences were also reported in a multiracial country like Malaysia, where the prevalence of reflux-type symptoms was more common among Indians (7.5%; 95% CI, 4.4–11.7) than Chinese (0.8%; 95% CI, 0.1–3.0) and Malays (3.0%; 95% CI, 1.2–6.1) [12]. Another study of the prevalence of heartburn in a multiracial population, based on a gastrointestinal symptoms questionnaire, showed that the annual prevalence of heartburn was more in Indians (42.4%) as compared to Chinese (29.3%) and Malays (29%). Indians vs. Chinese odds ratio 1.77; 95% CI, 1.26–2.50, $p < 0.001$; Indians vs. Malays OR 1.80; 95% CI, 1.28–2.54, $p < 0.001$ [13]. Similar differences were seen in the GERD complication rates.

The prevalence of heartburn was similar in Malays (mainly Muslims) and Chinese (mainly Buddhist or Christian), despite difference in their alcohol intake. But this study was limited by the inability to access differences in exposure to environmental factors, such as dietary fat consumption and the prevalence of *cag*A-positive *Helicobacter pylori (H. pylori)* infection. These differences necessitate further studies to establish a genetic and/or environmental etiology [2].

There seems to be an increase over time: the prevalence rate of reflux esophagitis on endoscopy in East Asia was 3.4–5.0% before 2000 and 4.3–15.7% after 2005 [14]. One time-trend study reported a significant increase in cases of esophagitis over a 10-year period among Indians (2.4–8.1%), Malays (1.5–3.7%), and Chinese (1.7–6.4%) [15]. There does not seem to be significant change in the prevalence of Barrett's esophagus in Asia over time.

In most Asian patients, GERD runs a benign course, with a majority of the patients having nonerosive reflux disease (NERD); progression from NERD to erosive esophagitis and complications is low [16, 17]. Complicated GERD appears to be more frequent in whites (12.3%), while only 2.8 and 4.8% of black and West Asian patients, respectively, had complicated GERD [16]. There was no GERD-related complication in any East Asian patient in one study [18].

Different Prevalence Rates in GERD Symptoms Due to Differences in Terminology?

Several explanations have been proposed for the reported differences in prevalence rates. These include the common suspects such as smaller body mass of Asians, lower basal as well as maximal gastric acid secretion, increased prevalence of *H. pylori* infection, low-fat Asian diet, and probably less use of alcohol and tobacco (the latter is debatable). Less well-recognized factors include the lack of a universal definition of GERD, lack of a word for heartburn in some languages, differences in physician recognition and diagnostic practices (e.g., reluctance to undergo endoscopy), and differences in referral patterns.

In the majority of prevalence studies, the diagnosis is symptom-based, using the presence of cardinal symptoms like heartburn and regurgitation as indicator of reflux disease. (This may also explain the differences in prevalence rates reported from the same population in different studies.) When heartburn or acid regurgitation dominates the patient's symptoms, they have very high specificity but low sensitivity for GERD [19]. Atypical or associated symptoms include noncardiac chest pain, acidic taste in the mouth, globus sensation, asthma, and bloating.

Heartburn is typically described as a burning sensation in the chest with discomfort, extending from the upper abdomen to the chest and sometimes to the jaw. As the name suggests, this symptom can easily be confused with cardiac chest pain. There is no word for heartburn in some languages spoken in Asia (Malay, Chinese, Korean, Tamil) [20]. One multiethnic study showed that, as compared to 35% of whites and 46% of blacks, only 3% of Asians complained of heartburn, and as compared to 35% of whites and 54% of blacks, only 13% of Asians understood heartburn appropriately [18]. Regurgitation is even more difficult to describe; in India, for example, in the absence of a single word in the multiple of dialects in the country, the physician needs to describe the sequence of events ("can you feel food or water or any content rising up from the abdomen, maybe even into the mouth?") to elicit understanding and response.

Probably because of language issues and perceptions, Asians seem to present more commonly with atypical symptoms as compared to the rest of the world; a distinction may be made in a clinic, but this is not easily possible in a field study. The lack of translated and validated questionnaires for the diagnosis of GERD makes it even more difficult.

Why the Rising Prevalence Rates?

Multiple environmental factors have been incriminated in the growing incidence of GERD in Asia. These include rising socioeconomic standards with consequent Westernization of lifestyle and diet (a predominantly carbohydrate-based diet to one that contains more protein and fat) and increase in BMI, increasing the use of alcohol and tobacco and presumably decreasing *H. pylori* prevalence (with consequent increase in gastric acid secretion). An increase in gastric acid secretion in the Japanese population since 1970 has been reported, unrelated to *H. pylori* infection; this may be secondary to increase in dietary fat intake [21]. Increased awareness of disease and improvement in available diagnostic techniques also could play a role. The contribution from stress in a more competitive society to the initiation or aggravation of symptoms of GERD has not been quantified.

Factors Impacting Pathophysiology

Although there is no strong reason to suspect that there would be differences in the basic pathophysiological factors for GERD between ethnic groups and regions, the fact remains that there are limited studies in this regard. Normal reference values for esophageal pH and manometry among racial groups are presently not available; this may be important considering the lower acid outputs recorded in Asian populations. Chinese patients with GERD who underwent esophageal manometry and 24-h ambulatory esophageal pH monitoring were no different from control subjects in the frequency of transient lower esophageal sphincter relaxation (TLESR), but had significantly lower successful primary peristalsis (59% vs. 70%, $p = 0.04$), suggesting impaired esophageal clearance by defective peristalsis [22]. Hiatal hernia is an infrequent finding in Asian GERD patients even in the presence of esophagitis [23, 24].

Obesity is an important risk factor for GERD. An independent association between increasing abdominal girth and GERD symptoms was identified in whites but not in blacks and Asians [25]. Another symptom-based study showed consistent association between abdominal girth (independent of BMI) and reflux-type symptoms in the white population but not in the black population or Asians [25]. A recent study found a homogeneous increase in GERD prevalence with increasing BMI in US studies, whereas studies from Europe provided heterogeneous results [26]. BMI cutoff points to define obesity and overweight are lower in Asian countries than those currently used in Western countries, but this may not be applicable to all ethnic groups. For the same body fat, African Americans had lower BMI (1.3 kg/m^2) as compared to Chinese (1.9), Thais (2.9), Indonesians (3.2), and Ethiopians (4.6) [27].

Factors Impacting Treatment

The current standard of medical care for the treatment of GERD is proton pump inhibitors (PPI). The principal enzyme involved in PPI metabolism is the cytochrome p450 isoform CYP2C19, the phenotypes of which are classified into extensive, intermediate, and poor metabolizers [28]. Studies on racial differences in CYP2C19 genotype polymorphism had shown a higher frequency of poor metabolizers among Asians (11–24%) as compared to 2–5% among whites [29]. Healing rate of erosive esophagitis was only 77% in extensive metabolizers as compared to 95 and 100% for intermediate and poor metabolizers, respectively ($p < 0.05$) [30]. CYP2C19 genotype was not found to be associated with reflux symptoms or esophageal acid exposure [31]. Although in clinical practice CYP2C19 genotype determination is unlikely to predict efficacy of a PPI, a recent study suggested that lower dose of PPI may be sufficient to control reflux symptoms in Asian populations with their lower acid secretory capacity [32]. In patients with severe esophagitis who are refractory to standard treatment, the possibility of their being extensive metabolizers should be considered.

Cultural Differences in Treatment: The Use of Complementary and Alternative Medicines

Complementary and alternative medicines are those that are not an integral part of conventional allopathic medical practice; their use in the treatment for GERD is probably more frequent in Asian regions where they have existed for centuries for treatment of all kinds of illnesses. One study reported that 6.7% of patients use alternative treatment for heartburn [13]. These include milk, peppermint, botanicals and mixtures of herbs, melatonin, yoga, acupuncture, magnet therapy, hypnosis, massage, and other relaxation techniques. Some of these are detailed below.

Yoga

Forms of yoga involving breathing control techniques (*pranayama*), like *kapalbhati* and *agnisar kriya*, increase diaphragmatic tone and thereby can decrease gastro-esophageal reflux. *Kapalbhati* involves passive inspiration and active expiration using abdominal muscles for clearance of the respiratory passage and strengthening the diaphragm [33]. *Agnisar kriya* is a method in which contracting or flapping of abdominal muscles in and out is believed to help digestion. Apart from increasing diaphragmatic tone, these maneuvers are believed to decrease TLESR and increase lower esophageal sphincter tone [24].

Another possible mechanism by which yoga works is impacting the autonomic nervous system via a relaxation response, which is associated with physiological changes in respiratory rate and lowering of heart rate and blood pressure mediated by reduction in epinephrine [34]. Stress-induced increase in gastric acid secretion may also be decreased in the relaxation phase of yoga [35].

Magnet Therapy

Magnetic bracelets, straps, and blankets, which involve the use of static magnetic fields, are an alternative treatment used for GERD. The LINX system, which is a ring of titanium beads with magnetic cores, connected together with titanium wires, was approved by the US FDA in 2012 for the treatment of refractory GERD [36].

Acupuncture

Acupuncture uses stainless steel needles on specific points along the body (acu-points) to rebalance energy flow; this has been used in traditional Chinese medicine for millennia. Electroacupuncture stimulates needles with an electrical current rather than manual manipulation. Acupuncture possibly works by inhibiting intraesophageal acid and bile reflux [37] as well as increasing LES pressure and reducing TLESR [38]. One study showed that adding acupuncture is more effective than doubling the PPI dose in controlling GERD-related symptoms in patients who failed standard-dose PPI [39].

Botanicals (Herbs)

Lonicera, the Chinese honeysuckle flower, has been evaluated in animal studies as a possible treatment for GERD. In one such study, rats given a preparation of the flower were found to have significant improvement in esophageal lesion scores and thickness of the esophageal mucous membrane [40]. Another product is Iberogast, made with nine herbs, including angelica, caraway, clown's mustard plant, German chamomile, greater celandine, lemon balm, licorice, milk thistle, and peppermint. Trials done earlier for evaluating its efficacy in patients with functional dyspepsia noted symptomatic improvement in the subgroup of patients with GERD-like symptoms [41]. The herbal product spearmint was reported to be useful in the treatment of heartburn, but failed in volunteers [42]. Peppermint oil enhances gastric emptying (especially in the early phase) and, while decreasing pressure in the resting LES, may be beneficial in GERD [42].

Melatonin

Melatonin is produced in the pineal gland, esophagus, and other parts of the GI tract. It has been shown to stimulate LES activity, which prevents acid-pepsin-induced esophagitis; it also protects the gut mucosa from oxidative damage caused by reactive oxygen species [43]. One small study involving 36 patients, to evaluate the role of exogenous melatonin alone or in combination with omeprazole in the treatment of reflux disease, showed that the combination therapy was preferable [44].

Milk

Milk can temporarily buffer stomach acid, although it can also stimulate acid production due to its fat content; its efficacy in the treatment of GERD has not been proven.

Conclusion

The multiethnic, multicultural spectrum of Asia makes it a suitable region for study of the role of these factors and diet on GERD prevalence, pathophysiology, and treatment. Unfortunately, there is a paucity of studies addressing these aspects from many parts of Asia, and available studies are largely from regions that in recent decades have had strong Western influences. Basic pathophysiological factors may be common with the West, but studies show differences in prevalence and intensity and recent time-trends changes. PPI is the standard of care for treatment of GERD in Asia, especially in institutes, but alternative treatment modalities are quite frequently in use.

References

1. El-Serag HB, Petersen NJ, Carter J, Graham DY, Richardson P, Genta RM, et al. Gastroesophageal reflux among different racial groups in the United States. Gastroenterology. 2004;126(7):1692–9.
2. Dent J, El-Serag HB, Wallander MA, Johansson S. Epidemiology of gastro-oesophageal reflux disease: a systematic review. Gut. 2005;54:710–7.
3. Ronkainen J, Agreus L. Epidemiology of reflux symptoms and GORD. Best Pract Res Clin Gastroenterol. 2013;27:325–37.
4. Bhatia SJ, Reddy DN, Ghoshal UC, Jayanthi V, Abraham P, Choudhuri G, et al. Epidemiology and symptom profile of gastroesophageal reflux in the Indian population: report of the Indian Society of Gastroenterology Task Force. Indian J Gastroenterol. 2011;30(3):118–27.
5. Sharma PK, Ahuja V, Madan K, Gupta S, Raizada A, Sharma MP. Prevalence, severity, and risk factors of symptomatic gastroesophageal reflux disease among employees of a large hospital in northern India. Indian J Gastroenterol. 2011;30:128–34.
6. Jafri N, Jafri W, Yakoob J, Islam M, Manzoor S, Jalil A, et al. Perception of gastroesophageal reflux disease in urban population in Pakistan. J Coll Physicians Surg Pak. 2005;15(9):532–4.
7. Lien HC, Chang CS, Yeh HZ, Ko CW, Chang HY, Cheng KF, et al. Increasing prevalence of erosive esophagitis among Taiwanese aged 40 years and above: a comparison between two time periods. J Clin Gastroenterol. 2009;43:926–32.
8. Wang JH, Luo JY, Dong L, Gong J, Tong M. Epidemiology of gastroesophageal reflux disease: a general population-based study in Xi'an of Northwest China. World J Gastroenterol. 2004;10:1647–51.
9. Wong WM, Lai KC, Lam KF, Hui WM, Hu WH, Lam CL, et al. Prevalence, clinical spectrum and health care utilization of gastro-oesophageal reflux disease in a Chinese population: a population-based study. Aliment Pharmacol Ther. 2003;18(6):595–604.
10. Rokonuzzaman SM, Bhuian MR, Ali MH, Paul GK, Khan MR, Mamun AA. Epidemiological study of gastro-esophageal reflux disease in rural population. Mymensingh Med J. 2011;20:463–71.
11. Mohammed I, Nightingale P, Trudgill NJ. Risk factors for gastro-oesophageal reflux disease symptoms: a community study. Aliment Pharmacol Ther. 2005;21:821–7.
12. Ho KY, Kang JY, Seow A. Prevalence of gastrointestinal symptoms in a multiracial Asian population, with particular reference to reflux-type symptoms. Am J Gastroenterol. 1998;93:1816–22.
13. Rajendra S, Alahuddin S. Racial differences in the prevalence of heartburn. Aliment Pharmacol Ther. 2004;19:375–6.
14. Jung HK. Epidemiology of gastroesophageal reflux disease in Asia: a systematic review. J Neurogastroenterol Motil. 2011;17:14–27.
15. Goh KL, Wong HT, Lim CH, Rosaida MS. Time trends in peptic ulcer, erosive reflux oesophagitis, gastric and oesophageal cancers in a multiracial Asian population. Aliment Pharmacol Therap. 2009;29:774–80.
16. Wu JC. Gastroesophageal reflux disease: an Asian perspective. J Gastroenterol Hepatol. 2008;23:1785–93.
17. Goh KL. Gastroesophageal reflux disease in Asia: a historical perspective and present challenges. J Gastroenterol Hepatol. 2011;26(Suppl 1):2–10.
18. Spechler SJ, Jain SK, Tendler DA, Parker RA. Racial differences in the frequency of symptoms and complications of gastro-oesophageal reflux disease. Aliment Pharmacol Ther. 2002;16:1795–800.
19. Klauser AG, Schindlbeck NE, Muller-Lissner SA. Symptoms in gastro-oesophageal reflux disease. Lancet. 1990;335:205–8.
20. Goh KL, Chang CS, Fock KM, Ke M, Park HJ, Lam SK. Gastro-oesophageal reflux disease in Asia. J Gastroenterol Hepatol. 2000;15:230–8.

21. Kinoshita Y, Kawanami C, Kishi K, Nakata H, Seino Y, Chiba T. *Helicobacter pylori*-independent chronological change in gastric acid secretion in the Japanese. Gut. 1997;41:452–8.
22. Wong WM, Lai KC, Hui WM, Hu WH, Huang JQ, Wong NY, et al. Pathophysiology of gastro-esophageal reflux diseases in Chinese--role of transient lower esophageal sphincter relaxation and esophageal motor dysfunction. Am J Gastroenterol. 2004;99:2088–93.
23. Rosaida MS, Goh KL. Gastro-oesophageal reflux disease, reflux oesophagitis and non-erosive reflux disease in a multiracial Asian population: a prospective, endoscopy based study. Eur J Gastroenterol Hepatol. 2004;16:495–501.
24. Yeh C, Hsu CT, Ho AS, Sampliner RE, Fass R. Erosive esophagitis and Barrett's esophagus in Taiwan: a higher frequency than expected. Dig Dis Sci. 1997;42(4):702–6.
25. Corley DA, Kubo A, Zhao W. Abdominal obesity, ethnicity and gastro-oesophageal reflux symptoms. Gut. 2007;56:756–62.
26. Corley DA, Kubo A. Body mass index and gastroesophageal reflux disease: a systematic review and meta-analysis. Am J Gastroenterol. 2006;101:2619–28.
27. Chang CJ, Wu CH, Chang CS, Yao WJ, Yang YC, Wu JS, et al. Low body mass index but high percent body fat in Taiwanese subjects: implications of obesity cutoffs. Int J Obes Relat Metab Disord. 2003;27(2):253–9.
28. Klotz U, Schwab M, Treiber G. CYP2C19 polymorphism and proton pump inhibitors. Basic Clin Pharmacol Toxicol. 2004;95:2–8.
29. Lim PW, Goh KL, Wong BC. CYP2C19 genotype and the PPIs--focus on rabeprazole. J Gastroenterol Hepatol. 2005;20(Suppl):S22–8.
30. Kawamura M, Ohara S, Koike T, Iijima K, Suzuki J, Kayaba S, et al. The effects of lansoprazole on erosive reflux oesophagitis are influenced by CYP2C19 polymorphism. Aliment Pharmacol Ther. 2003;17(7):965–73.
31. Egan LJ, Myhre GM, Mays DC, Dierkhising RA, Kammer PP, Murray JA. CYP2C19 pharmacogenetics in the clinical use of proton-pump inhibitors for gastro-oesophageal reflux disease: variant alleles predict gastric acid suppression, but not oesophageal acid exposure or reflux symptoms. Aliment Pharmacol Ther. 2003;17:1521–8.
32. Wong WM, Lai KC, Hui WM, Lam KF, Huang JQ, Hu WH, et al. Double-blind, randomized controlled study to assess the effects of lansoprazole 30 mg and lansoprazole 15 mg on 24-h oesophageal and intragastric pH in Chinese subjects with gastro-oesophageal reflux disease. Aliment Pharmacol Ther. 2004;19:455–62.
33. Kaswala D, Shah S, Mishra A, Patel H, Patel N, Sangwan P, et al. Can yoga be used to treat gastroesophageal reflux disease? Int J Yoga. 2013;6:131–3.
34. Benson H. Hypnosis and the relaxation response. Gastroenterology. 1989;96:1609–11.
35. Goldman MC. Gastric secretion during a medical interview. Psychosom Med. 1963;25:351–6.
36. Ganz RA, Peters JH, Horgan S, Bemelman WA, Dunst CM, Edmundowicz SA, et al. Esophageal sphincter device for gastroesophageal reflux disease. N Engl J Med. 2013;368(8):719–27.
37. Zhang CX, Qin YM, Guo BR. Clinical study on the treatment of gastroesophageal reflux by acupuncture. Chin J Integr Med. 2010;16:298–303.
38. Zou D, Chen WH, Iwakiri K, Rigda R, Tippett M, Holloway RH. Inhibition of transient lower esophageal sphincter relaxations by electrical acupoint stimulation. Am J Physiol Gastrointest Liver Physiol. 2005;289:G197–201.
39. Dickman R, Schiff E, Holland A, Wright C, Sarela SR, Han B, et al. Clinical trial: acupuncture vs. doubling the proton pump inhibitor dose in refractory heartburn. Aliment Pharmacol Ther. 2007;26:1333–44.
40. Ku SK, Seo BI, Park JH, Park GY, Seo YB, Kim JS, et al. Effect of Lonicerae Flos extracts on reflux esophagitis with antioxidant activity. World J Gastroenterol. 2009;15:4799–805.
41. Patrick L. Gastroesophageal reflux disease (GERD): a review of conventional and alternative treatments. Alt Med Rev. 2011;16:116–33.
42. Bulat R, Fachnie E, Chauhan U, Chen Y, Tougas G. Lack of effect of spearmint on lower oesophageal sphincter function and acid reflux in healthy volunteers. Aliment Pharmacol Ther. 1999;13:805–12.

43. Reiter RJ, Tan DX, Mayo JC, Sainz RM, Leon J, Czarnocki Z. Melatonin as an antioxidant: biochemical mechanisms and pathophysiological implications in humans. Acta Biochim Polonica. 2003;50:1129–46.
44. Kandil TS, Mousa AA, El-Gendy AA, Abbas AM. The potential therapeutic effect of melatonin in gastro-esophageal reflux disease. BMC Gastroenterol. 2010;10:7.

Srinivas Gaddam and Prateek Sharma

Abstract

Until recently, GERD was thought to be a rare disease in Asia, and research on this topic was sparse. Now several publications have evaluated the prevalence of reflux symptoms in the Asian population. These large studies have predominantly been from China, Korea, Japan, Turkey, Iran, and Israel and show the incidence of GERD is rising throughout Asia.

Keywords

Gastroesophageal reflux disease • Barrett's esophagus • Low-grade dysplasia • High-grade dysplasia • Endoscopy • Endoscopic ablation • Endoscopic mucosal resection • Advanced imaging

Introduction

Until recently, gastroesophageal reflux disease (GERD) was thought to be a rare disease in Asia [1–3]. Several diseases of the gastrointestinal tract have been shown to have increasing incidences in India. Crohn's disease was thought to be nonexistent in the latter part of the twentieth century in India. However, there is accumulating data now that the incidence is steeply higher than previously thought [4]. A recent study by Mathew et al. found that the incidence of Barrett's esophagus is not uncommon in India [5]. Similarly, recent studies have shown a rising incidence of

S. Gaddam
Department of Gastroenterology and Hepatology, Veterans Affairs Medical Center,
4801 E. Linwood Blvd, Kansas City, MO 64128-2295, USA

P. Sharma (✉)
University of Kansas School of Medicine, VA Medical Center, Kansas City, MO, USA
e-mail: psharma@kumc.edu

© Springer India 2018
P. Sharma et al. (eds.), *The Rise of Acid Reflux in Asia*,
DOI 10.1007/978-81-322-0846-4_13

GERD in India [3, 6–9]. Whether these increases are due to improved recognition and access to better diagnostic tools or a true increase in the prevalence is unclear [10].

GERD is a well-studied disease in the western world. Based on population-based data, at least 20% of the general population experiences heartburn and/or regurgitation weekly [11]. It is the most common gastrointestinal disease and is associated with a significant decrease in quality of life and is a huge economic burden [2, 12–16]. In the USA, GERD accounts for $10 billion in direct costs and up to $75 billion in indirect costs per year [13, 14]. Moreover, uncontrolled GERD can result in complications such as strictures, Barrett's esophagus, and esophageal adenocarcinoma (EAC) [17–19].

Status of Research on GERD in Asia

Contrary to the western world, research on this topic in Asia was sparse until recently, and GERD was considered to be uncommon in this part of the world [1]. However, now several publications have evaluated the prevalence of reflux symptoms in the Asian population [1]. These large studies have predominantly been from China, Korea, Japan, Turkey, Iran, and Israel. Three large studies from China, based on a symptom questionnaire and each with more than 2500 patients, estimated the prevalence of GERD (defined as at least once-a-week symptoms of heartburn and/ or regurgitation) to be 2.5–4.8% [16, 20–22]. Large studies out of Korea ($n = 1902$) and Japan ($n = 6035$) have reported similar prevalence rates of 3.5% and 6.6%, respectively [23, 24]. Western and southern Asia have reported much higher prevalence of GERD [25, 26]. Bor et al. from Turkey report a prevalence of 20% using face-to-face interviews utilizing the Gastroesophageal Reflux Questionnaire (GERQ) [25]. Similar studies from Iran and Israel report a GERD prevalence of 21.2% and 9.3%, respectively [26, 27]. Whether these geographic differences in prevalence of GERD are due to variations in study design or due to other cultural and ethnic differences is unclear. An interesting study by Ho et al. based on a multiracial population in Singapore suggests that this variation is likely due to racial differences [28]. They report GERD prevalence of 7.5% among Indians compared to a low prevalence of 0.8% among Chinese. Nonetheless, there is emerging data that the incidence and prevalence of GERD continue to rise [29].

Research on GERD has been scarce in India. Therefore, in 2011, the Indian Society of Gastroenterology formed a task force to study the prevalence and risk factors for GERD. Bhatia et al. studied 3224 urban and rural adult populations and found that the prevalence of GERD was 7.6% and that consumption of nonvegetarian food was an independent risk factor for GERD [6]. Another study by Sharma et al. found that the GERD was present in 16.2% of 4039 employees of a tertiary care center [8]. They found that high BMI, smoking, asthma, and hypertension were independent risk factors for the development of GERD. Finally, a study by Kumar et al. reported a prevalence of 18.7% while studying 905 adult patients [7]. They found that younger age, sedentary lifestyle, serum LDL of more than 150 mg/dL, high consumption of meat, and low consumption of tea and fresh fruits were independent risk factors for GERD. These studies had varying definitions and methodology. Nonetheless, they are the first large-scale evaluations of burden of disease of GERD in India and draw our attention to a high prevalence that is comparable to the western world.

The complications of chronic GERD have received much less attention in Asia. This is likely due to the initial data showing a much lower prevalence of reflux esophagitis and Barrett's esophagus in Asia when compared to the western world [29]. Low prevalence of erosive esophagitis was reported (5.6–16.8%) in patients undergoing an endoscopy [30–37]. Similarly, most studies have suggested a low prevalence of Barrett's esophagus (0.06–0.22% in general population and 0.5–2% in symptomatic patients) in Asia [38–42]. However, newer studies show that the prevalence of BE in symptomatic GERD patients (7.4–9%) is likely higher than previously reported [5, 37]. The data on incidence and time trends in esophageal adenocarcinoma from Asia are also unclear. There appear to be an increasing trend in Japan and Singapore, no change in Hong Kong, but a decreasing trend in Taiwan and Korea [43–47]. Data is almost nonexistent on this topic from other parts of Asia. These studies on complications of GERD show contrasting results, but even so, they draw attention to the paucity of data regarding Barrett's esophagus and esophageal adenocarcinoma from Asia.

Challenges and Future Directions to GERD Research in Asia

Healthcare Disparities

There are several challenges to conducting research in Asia due to its multilingual, multiethnic, and multicultural variations. There are several plausible explanations for these differences in epidemiology. Most studies are performed on patients seeking medical care. Due to variations in the structure of healthcare finance and delivery across different countries, there are wide disparities in equity and access to gastroenterologists and endoscopy suites. In addition, there are also variations to physician recognition, diagnostic practices, and referral patterns. These issues can result in the study of a biased patient group, resulting in confounded results. Therefore, large population-based studies are needed to understand the true epidemiology of GERD. Future research should also focus on understanding health behaviors such as healthcare-seeking behaviors, adherence to medical advice, and compliance to medications.

Language Barriers

GERD is a symptom-based diagnosis and does not have a gold standard test. GERD is evaluated in most studies by using patient-response symptom questionnaires that were validated in the western world. Most times, the translations of these questionnaires have not been validated. In some languages such as Chinese, Malay, and

Korean, there is no direct representative term for heartburn. This can severely impair the validity of the study results. Therefore, culturally acceptable and validated GERD questionnaires in a local language should be used as an instrument for diagnosis.

Economic Inequalities

Asia has experienced economic inequalities and very disparate growth rates. On one hand, there are countries that have showed rapid growth and attained the status of developed countries over three or four decades (four Asian tigers—Singapore, Hong Kong, South Korea, and Taiwan), while on the other hand, there are several countries below the poverty line. This results in wide dissimilarities in education and access to healthcare. Even within each country, there are significant dissimilarities between the urban and rural populations. This limits the generalizability of any study and more so studies on GERD. It is suggested that the increase in GERD may be related to urbanization, improvement in socioeconomic status, and adaptation of a western lifestyle [29]. Therefore, the prevalence outcomes may be profoundly affected by the geographic location of its participants. Future studies should attempt to include diverse populations while studying GERD. A stratified analysis by geographic location, level of education, and socioeconomic status may be warranted to better understand the influence of each of these factors on GERD.

Extraesophageal GERD Symptoms and Complications

There are limited data on extraesophageal GERD symptoms. Future studies must utilize other diagnostic studies, such as pH-impedance studies, to better evaluate extraesophageal symptoms where applicable. In addition, complications of GERD such as stricture rates, Barrett's esophagus, and esophageal adenocarcinoma need to be evaluated. These potentially preventable complications can have profound impact on costs, health-related quality of life, and morbidity. Research on true prevalence and data on outcomes on therapy of extraesophageal symptoms and complications of GERD can guide policy-makers on suitable allocations of healthcare resources.

Efficacy of Therapy for GERD

GERD is chronic disorder that requires long-term acid suppression therapy [48]. Proton pump inhibitors (PPI) are considered the gold standard treatment for GERD. Previous studies have shown high healing rates of erosive esophagitis in the Asian population [49]. While it has been shown that GERD phenotypes of nonerosive reflux esophagitis and erosive esophagitis are not categorical diseases in the western population, this has never been evaluated in the Asian population. Furthermore, the role of *H. pylori* and its influence on PPI therapy are unclear. It has been suggested that PPI therapy in patients who harbor *H. pylori* is likely to progress to atrophic gastritis [50]. Future studies should evaluate for the role of these potential risk factors and confounders in the management of GERD.

Conclusion

GERD is an extremely common GI disease and is associated with poor health-related quality of life and is a huge financial burden. The current status of research on GERD, its complications, and management are not well studied in the Asian population. The diverse nature of Asian countries with regard to cultural beliefs, socioeconomic status, health equity, access, and delivery makes for a challenging environment for research studies. Well-designed studies on all aspects of GERD, listed below, are needed to help with effective management of GERD patients and, in addition, to provide policy-makers with data to help with allocation of healthcare resources.

Directions for Future Research on GERD in Asia

1. Consensus on a common definition of GERD
2. Determination of incidence and prevalence of GERD and extraesophageal symptoms of GERD
3. Determination of incidence and prevalence of complications of GERD (strictures, Barrett's esophagus, and esophageal adenocarcinoma)
4. Separation of true GERD from functional heartburn, peptic ulcer disease, and functional dyspepsia
5. Evaluation of effects of GERD on health-related quality of life
6. Culturally apt translations of existing questionnaires and validation of these instruments
7. Population-based studies to account for inequity and lack of access to healthcare resources
8. Endoscopy, pH-impedance, and manometry-based studies to help with accurate diagnosis
9. Interaction between *H. pylori* infection and GERD symptoms
10. Delineation of risk factors for GERD and its complications
11. Evaluation of efficacy and role of medical and surgical therapy for GERD
12. Comparative efficacy of therapeutic agents for GERD
13. Role and efficacy of non-pharmacologic therapy for GERD
14. Qualitative research on health behaviors such as healthcare-seeking behaviors, adherence to medical advice, and compliance to medications
15. Assessment of physician knowledge and training with regard to GERD and its complications
16. Identification of health education techniques and evaluation of efficacy of education program

17. Long-term outcomes of GERD and its complications
18. Identification of potential causes and confounders that predispose patients to GERD in the Asian population
19. Evaluation for pathophysiologic differences and pharmacokinetic variations based on ethnicity and geographic location
20. Assessment of influence of changes in socioeconomic status, changes in diet, and urbanization on the prevalence of GERD

References

1. Sharma P, Wani S, Romero Y, Johnson D, Hamilton F. Racial and geographic issues in gastro-esophageal reflux disease. Am J Gastroenterol. 2008;103(11):2669–80. doi:10.1111/j.1572-0241.2008.02089.x. Epub 2008 Nov 27. PMID: 19032462
2. Dent J, El-Serag HB, Wallander MA, Johansson S. Epidemiology of gastro-oesophageal reflux disease: a systematic review. Gut. 2005;54(5):710–7. doi:10.1136/gut.2004.051821. Epub 2005 Apr 16. PMID: 15831922; PMCID: PMC1774487
3. Ho KY. From GERD to Barrett's esophagus: is the pattern in Asia mirroring that in the west? J Gastroenterol Hepatol. 2011;26(5):816–24. doi:10.1111/j.1440-1746.2011.06669.x. Epub 2011 Jan 27. PMID: 21265879
4. Desai HG, Gupte PA. Increasing incidence of Crohn's disease in India: is it related to improved sanitation? Indian J Gastroenterol. 2005;24(1):23–4. Epub 2005 Mar 22. PMID: 15778522.
5. Mathew P, Joshi AS, Shukla A, Bhatia SJ. Risk factors for Barrett's esophagus in Indian patients with gastroesophageal reflux disease. J Gastroenterol Hepatol. 2011;26(7):1151–6. doi:10.1111/j.1440-1746.2011.06714.x. Epub 2011 Mar 8. PMID: 21375585
6. Bhatia SJ, Reddy DN, Ghoshal UC, Jayanthi V, Abraham P, Choudhuri G, et al. Epidemiology and symptom profile of gastroesophageal reflux in the Indian population: report of the Indian Society of Gastroenterology Task Force. Indian J Gastroenterol. 2011;30(3):118–27.
7. Kumar S, Sharma S, Norboo T, Dolma D, Norboo A, Stobdan T, et al. Population based study to assess prevalence and risk factors of gastroesophageal reflux disease in a high altitude area. Indian J Gastroenterol. 2011;30(3):135–43. doi:10.1007/s12664-010-0066-4. Epub 2010 Dec 25. PMID: 21181325
8. Sharma PK, Ahuja V, Madan K, Gupta S, Raizada A, Sharma MP. Prevalence, severity, and risk factors of symptomatic gastroesophageal reflux disease among employees of a large hospital in northern India. Indian J Gastroenterol. 2011;30(3):128–34. doi:10.1007/s12664-010-0065-5. Epub 2010 Nov 10. PMID: 21061110
9. Ramu B. Mohan P. Jayanthi V. Prevalence and risk factors for gastroesophageal reflux in pregnancy. Indian J Gastroenterol: Rajasekaran MS; 2010. doi:10.1007/s12664-010-0067-3. Epub 2010 Jan 3. PMID: 21125366
10. Gaddam S, Sharma P. Shedding light on the epidemiology of gastroesophageal reflux disease in India--a big step forward. Indian J Gastroenterol. 2011;30(3):105–7. doi:10.1007/s12664-011-0108-6. Epub 2011 Jul 26. PMID: 21785993
11. Locke GR 3rd, Talley NJ, Fett SL, Zinsmeister AR, Melton LJ 3rd. Prevalence and clinical spectrum of gastroesophageal reflux: a population-based study in Olmsted County, Minnesota. Gastroenterology. 1997;112(5):1448–56. PMID: 9136821
12. Kahrilas PJ. Clinical practice. Gastroesophageal reflux disease. N Engl J Med. 2008;359(16):1700–7. doi:10.1056/NEJMcp0804684. Epub 2008 Oct 17. PMID: 18923172
13. Shaheen NJ, Hansen RA, Morgan DR, Gangarosa LM, Ringel Y, Thiny MT, et al. The burden of gastrointestinal and liver diseases, 2006. Am J Gastroenterol. 2006;101(9):2128–38. doi:10.1111/j.1572-0241.2006.00723.x. Epub 2006 Jul 20. PMID: 16848807

14. Wahlqvist P, Reilly MC, Barkun A. Systematic review: the impact of gastro-oesophageal reflux disease on work productivity. Aliment Pharmacol Ther. 2006;24(2):259–72. doi:10.1111/j.1365-2036.2006.02996.x. Epub 2006 Jul 18. PMID: 16842452

15. El-Serag HB. Time trends of gastroesophageal reflux disease: a systematic review. Clin Gastroenterol Hepatol. 2007;5(1):17–26. doi: S1542-3565(06)00944-X10.1016/j. cgh.2006.09.016. Epub 2006 Jan 5. PMID: 17142109

16. Wong BC, Kinoshita Y. Systematic review on epidemiology of gastroesophageal reflux disease in Asia. Clin Gastroenterol Hepatol. 2006;4(4):398–407. doi:10.1016/j.cgh.2005.10.011. Epub 2006 Apr 18. PMID: 16616342

17. Sharma P. Clinical practice. Barrett's esophagus. N Engl J Med. 2009;361(26):2548–56. doi: 361/26/254810.1056/NEJMcp0902173. Epub 2009 Dec 25. PMID: 20032324

18. Lagergren J, Bergstrom R, Lindgren A, Nyren O. Symptomatic gastroesophageal reflux as a risk factor for esophageal adenocarcinoma. N Engl J Med. 1999;340(11):825–31. doi:10.1056/NEJM199903183401101. Epub 1999 Mar 18. PMID: 10080844

19. Spechler SJ, Souza RF. Barrett's esophagus. N Engl J Med. 2014;371(9):836–45. doi:10.1056/NEJMra1314704. Epub 2014 Aug 28. PMID: 25162890

20. Wong WM, Lai KC, Lam KF, Hui WM, Hu WH, Lam CL, et al. Prevalence, clinical spectrum and health care utilization of gastro-oesophageal reflux disease in a Chinese population: a population-based study. Aliment Pharmacol Ther. 2003;18(6):595–604. Epub 2003 Sep 13. PMID: 12969086

21. Hu WH, Wong WM, Lam CL, Lam KF, Hui WM, Lai KC, et al. Anxiety but not depression determines health care-seeking behaviour in Chinese patients with dyspepsia and irritable bowel syndrome: a population-based study. Aliment Pharmacol Ther. 2002;16(12):2081–8. Epub 2002 Nov 28. PMID: 12452941

22. Guozong P, Guoming X, Meiyun K, Shaomei H, Huiping G, Zhaoshen L, et al. Epidemiological study of symptomatic gastroesophageal reflux disease in China: Beijing and shanghai. Chinese J Dig Dis. 2000;1(1):2–8. doi:10.1046/j.1443-9573.2000.00001.x.

23. Cho YS, Choi MG, Jeong JJ, Chung WC, Lee IS, Kim SW, et al. Prevalence and clinical spectrum of gastroesophageal reflux: a population-based study in Asan-si. Korea Am J Gastroenterol. 2005;100(4):747–53. doi:10.1111/j.1572–0241.2005.41245.x. Epub 2005 Mar 24. PMID: 15784014

24. Fujiwara Y, Higuchi K, Watanabe Y, Shiba M, Watanabe T, Tominaga K, et al. Prevalence of gastroesophageal reflux disease and gastroesophageal reflux disease symptoms in Japan. J Gastroenterol Hepatol. 2005;20(1):26–9. doi:10.1111/j.1440–1746.2004.03521.x. Epub 2004 Dec 22. PMID: 15610442

25. Bor S, Mandiracioglu A, Kitapcioglu G, Caymaz-Bor C, Gilbert RJ. Gastroesophageal reflux disease in a low-income region in Turkey. Am J Gastroenterol. 2005;100(4):759–65. doi:10.1111/j.1572–0241.2005.41065.x. Epub 2005 Mar 24. PMID: 15784016

26. Nouraie M, Radmard AR, Zaer-Rezaii H, Razjouyan H, Nasseri-Moghaddam S, Malekzadeh R. Hygiene could affect GERD prevalence independently: a population-based study in Tehran. Am J Gastroenterol. 2007;102(7):1353–60. doi:10.1111/j.1572–0241.2007.01208.x. Epub 2007 Apr 18. PMID: 17437507

27. Sperber AD, Halpern Z, Shvartzman P, Friger M, Freud T, Neville A, et al. Prevalence of GERD symptoms in a representative Israeli adult population. J Clin Gastroenterol. 2007;41(5):457–61. doi:10.1097/01.mcg.0000225664.68920.96. Epub 2007 Apr 24. PMID: 17450026

28. Ho KY, Kang JY, Seow A. Prevalence of gastrointestinal symptoms in a multiracial Asian population, with particular reference to reflux-type symptoms. American J Gastroenterol. 1998;93(10):1816–22. doi:10.1111/j.1572-0241.1998.00526.x. Epub 1998 Oct 15. PMID: 9772037

29. Wu JC. Gastroesophageal reflux disease: an Asian perspective. J Gastroenterol Hepatol. 2008;23(12):1785–93. doi:10.1111/j.1440-1746.2008.05684.x. Epub 2009 Jan 6. PMID: 19120871

30. Khuroo MS, Mahajan R, Zargar SA, Javid G, Munshi S. Prevalence of peptic ulcer in India: an endoscopic and epidemiological study in urban Kashmir. Gut. 1989;30(7):930–4. Epub 1989 Jul 1. PMID: 2788113; PMCID: PMC1434311

31. Kang JY, Tay HH, Yap I, Guan R, Lim KP, Math MV. Low frequency of endoscopic esophagitis in Asian patients. J Clin Gastroenterol. 1993;16(1):70–3. Epub 1993 Jan 01. PMID: 8421153

32. Rosaida MS, Goh KL. Gastro-oesophageal reflux disease, reflux oesophagitis and non-erosive reflux disease in a multiracial Asian population: a prospective, endoscopy based study. Eur J Gastroenterol Hepatol. 2004;16(5):495–501. Epub 2004 Apr 21. PMID: 15097043

33. Yeh C, Hsu CT, Ho AS, Sampliner RE, Fass R. Erosive esophagitis and Barrett's esophagus in Taiwan: a higher frequency than expected. Dig Dis Sci. 1997;42(4):702–6. Epub 1997 Apr 1. PubMed PMID: 9125635

34. Yeom JS, Park HJ, Cho JS, Lee SI, Park IS. Reflux esophagitis and its relationship to hiatal hernia. J Korean Med Sci. 1999;14(3):253–6. Epub 1999 Jul 13. PMID: 10402166; PMCID: PMC3054374

35. Furukawa N, Iwakiri R, Koyama T, Okamoto K, Yoshida T, Kashiwagi Y, et al. Proportion of reflux esophagitis in 6010 Japanese adults: prospective evaluation by endoscopy. J Gastroenterol. 1999;34(4):441–4. Epub 1999 Aug 19. PMID: 10452674

36. Inamori M, Togawa J, Nagase H, Abe Y, Umezawa T, Nakajima A, et al. Clinical characteristics of Japanese reflux esophagitis patients as determined by Los Angeles classification. J Gastroenterol Hepatol. 2003;18(2):172–6. Epub 2003 Jan 25 PMID: 12542602

37. Toruner M, Soykan I, Ensari A, Kuzu I, Yurdaydin C, Ozden A. Barrett's esophagus: prevalence and its relationship with dyspeptic symptoms. J Gastroenterol Hepatol. 2004;19(5):535–40. doi:10.1111/j.1440-1746.2003.03342.x. Epub 2004 Apr 17. PMID: 15086597

38. Park JJ, Kim JW, Kim HJ, Chung MG, Park SM, Baik GH, et al. The prevalence of and risk factors for Barrett's esophagus in a Korean population: a nationwide multicenter prospective study. J Clin Gastroenterol. 2009;43(10):907–14. doi:10.1097/MCG.0b013e318196bd11. Epub 2009 May 7. PMID: 19417682

39. Lee IS, Choi SC, Shim KN, Jee SR, Huh KC, Lee JH, et al. Prevalence of Barrett's esophagus remains low in the Korean population: nationwide cross-sectional prospective multicenter study. Dig Dis Sci. 2010;55(7):1932–9. doi:10.1007/s10620-009-0984-0. Epub 2009 Oct 3. PMID: 19798574.

40. Lee HS, Jeon SW. Barrett esophagus in Asia: same disease with different pattern. Clin Endosc. 2014;47(1):15–22. doi:10.5946/ce.2014.47.1.15. Epub 2014 Feb 27. PMID: 24570879; PMCID: PMC3928486

41. Tseng PH, Lee YC, Chiu HM, Huang SP, Liao WC, Chen CC, et al. Prevalence and clinical characteristics of Barrett's esophagus in a Chinese general population. J Clin Gastroenterol. 2008;42(10):1074–9. doi:10.1097/MCG.0b013e31809e7126. Epub 2008 Mar 25. PMID: 18360296

42. Wong WM, Lam SK, Hui WM, Lai KC, Chan CK, Hu WH, et al. Long-term prospective follow-up of endoscopic oesophagitis in southern Chinese--prevalence and spectrum of the disease. Aliment Pharmacol Ther. 2002;16(12):2037–42. Epub 2002 Nov 28. PMID: 12452935

43. Hongo M. Review article: Barrett's oesophagus and carcinoma in Japan. Aliment Pharmacol Ther. 2004;20(Suppl 8):50–4. doi:10.1111/j.1365-2036.2004.02230.x. Epub 2004 Dec 4. PMID: 15575874

44. Fernandes ML, Seow A, Chan YH, Ho KY. Opposing trends in incidence of esophageal squamous cell carcinoma and adenocarcinoma in a multi-ethnic Asian country. Am J Gastroenterol. 2006;101(7):1430–6. doi:10.1111/j.1572-0241.2006.00570.x. Epub 2006 Jul 26. PMID: 16863543

45. Yee YK, Cheung TK, Chan AO, Yuen MF, Wong BC. Decreasing trend of esophageal adenocarcinoma in Hong Kong. Cancer Epidemiol Biomark Prev. 2007;16(12):2637–40. doi:10.1158/1055-9965.EPI-07-0421. Epub 2007 Dec 19. PMID: 18086768

46. Chung JW, Lee GH, Choi KS, Kim DH, Jung KW, Song HJ, et al. Unchanging trend of esophagogastric junction adenocarcinoma in Korea: experience at a single institution

based on Siewert's classification. Dis Esophagus. 2009;22(8):676–81. doi:10.1111/j.1442-2050.2009.00946.x. Epub 2009 Feb 13. PMID: 19222529

47. Lu CL, Lang HC, Luo JC, Liu CC, Lin HC, Chang FY, et al. Increasing trend of the incidence of esophageal squamous cell carcinoma, but not adenocarcinoma, in Taiwan. Cancer Causes Control. 2010;21(2):269–74. doi:10.1007/s10552-009-9458-0. Epub 2009 Oct 29. PMID: 19866363

48. Nocon M, Labenz J, Jaspersen D, Meyer-Sabellek W, Stolte M, Lind T, et al. Long-term treatment of patients with gastro-oesophageal reflux disease in routine care - results from the ProGERD study. Aliment Pharmacol Ther. 2007;25(6):715–22. doi:10.1111/j.1365-2036.2007.03249.x. PMID: ISI:000245173000009

49. Wong WM, Lai KC, Hui WM, Lam KF, Huang JQ, Hu WH, et al. Double-blind, randomized controlled study to assess the effects of lansoprazole 30 mg and lansoprazole 15 mg on 24-h oesophageal and intragastric pH in Chinese subjects with gastro-oesophageal reflux disease. Aliment Pharmacol Ther. 2004;19(4):455–62. Epub 2004 Feb 12. PubMed PMID: 14871286

50. Kuipers EJ, Nelis GF, Klinkenberg-Knol EC, Snel P, Goldfain D, Kolkman JJ, et al. Cure of Helicobacter pylori infection in patients with reflux oesophagitis treated with long term omeprazole reverses gastritis without exacerbation of reflux disease: results of a randomised controlled trial. Gut. 2004;53(1):12–20. Epub 2003 Dec 20. PMID: 14684569; PMCID: PMC1773939